Case Studies in Neuropalliative Care

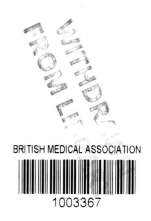

Case Studies in Neuropalliative Care

Edited by

Maisha T. Robinson, MD, MS

Mayo Clinic, Jacksonville, Florida

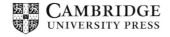

CAMBRIDGE
UNIVERSITY PRESS

CAMBRIDGE
UNIVERSITY PRESS

University Printing House, Cambridge CB2 8BS, United Kingdom

One Liberty Plaza, 20th Floor, New York, NY 10006, USA

477 Williamstown Road, Port Melbourne, VIC 3207, Australia

314–321, 3rd Floor, Plot 3, Splendor Forum, Jasola District Centre, New Delhi – 110025, India

79 Anson Road, #06–04/06, Singapore 079906

Cambridge University Press is part of the University of Cambridge.

It furthers the University's mission by disseminating knowledge in the pursuit of
education, learning, and research at the highest international levels of excellence.

www.cambridge.org
Information on this title: www.cambridge.org/9781108404914
DOI: 10.1017/9781108277365

© Cambridge University Press 2018

First published 2018

Printed in the United Kingdom by TJ International Ltd. Padstow Cornwall

A catalogue record for this publication is available from the British Library.

Library of Congress Cataloging-in-Publication Data
Names: Robinson, Maisha T., editor.
Title: Case studies in neuropalliative care / edited by Maisha T. Robinson, Mayo Clinic, Jacksonville, FL.
Description: Cambridge, United Kingdom ; New York, NY : Cambridge University Press, [2018] | Includes
bibliographical references and index.
Identifiers: LCCN 2017054569 | ISBN 9781108404914 (paperback : alk. paper)
Subjects: LCSH: Palliative treatment – Psychological aspects – Case studies. | Psychotherapy – Case studies.
Classification: LCC R726.8 .C3978 2018 | DDC 616.02/9–dc23
LC record available at https://lccn.loc.gov/2017054569

ISBN 978-1-108-40491-4 Paperback

....

Contents

Contributors

Jessica Besbris, MD
Department of Supportive Care Medicine
Department of Neurology
Cedars-Sinai Medical Center
Los Angeles, CA, USA

Alan Carver, MD
Department of Neurology
Memorial Sloan Kettering Cancer
Center
New York, NY, USA

Kristen Chasteen, MD
Section of Palliative Medicine
Henry Ford Health System
Detroit, MI, USA

William P. Cheshire Jr., MD, MA
Department of Neurology
Mayo Clinic
Jacksonville, FL, USA

Kimberly Chow, APRN
Supportive Care Service
Memorial Sloan Kettering Cancer
Center
New York, NY, USA

Claire J. Creutzfeldt, MD
Department of Neurology
Harborview Medical Center
Seattle, WA, USA

Gabriele C. DeLuca, MD, DPhil
Nuffield Department of Clinical
Neurosciences
University of Oxford
Oxford, UK

Jennifer E. Fugate, DO
Division of Critical Care Neurology
Mayo Clinic
Rochester, MN, USA

Paul Glare, MBBS
Pain Medicine
University of Sydney
Sydney, Australia

Priscilla H. Howick, MDiv
Chaplain Services
Mayo Clinic
Jacksonville, FL, USA

Joseph J. Hutchinson, BM, BCh
Oxford Medical School
University of Oxford
Oxford, UK

Benzi M. Kluger, MD, MS
Department of Neurology
University of Colorado School of
Medicine
Aurora, CO, USA

Neha M. Kramer, MD
Rush University Medical Center
Department of Neurology
Department of Internal Medicine, Section of
Palliative Medicine
Chicago, IL, USA

A. Sebastian Lopez Chiriboga, MD
Department of Neurology
Mayo Clinic
Rochester, MN, USA

Janis M. Miyasaki, MD, MEd
Division of Neurology
University of Alberta
Edmonton, Alberta, Canada

Sue E. Morris, PsyD
Psychosocial Oncology and Palliative
Care
Dana-Farber Cancer Institute
Boston, MA, USA

Kathryn Nevel, MD
Department of Neurology
Memorial Sloan Kettering Cancer Center
New York, NY, USA

Lauren K. Ng, MD, MPH
Department of Critical Care Medicine
Neurology and Neurosurgery
Mayo Clinic
Jacksonville, FL, USA

David J. Oliver, BSc, MBBS
Tizard Centre, University of Kent
Canterbury, Kent, UK

Daniel K. Partain, MD
Department of Internal Medicine
Mayo Clinic
Rochester, MN, USA

Joel Phillips, DO
Palliative and Supportive Care
Mercy Health Saint Mary's Hospital
Grand Rapids, MI, USA

Shayna Rich, MD, PhD
Haven Hospice
Lake City, FL, USA

Maisha T. Robinson, MD, MS
Department of Neurology
Palliative Medicine Service
Mayo Clinic
Jacksonville, FL, USA

Alva Roche-Green, MD
Department of Family Medicine
Palliative Medicine Service

Mayo Clinic
Jacksonville, FL, USA

Ugur Sener, MD
Department of Neurology
Mayo Clinic
Jacksonville, FL, USA

Imran Shariff, MD
Cancer Treatment Centers of America
Eastern Regional Medical Center
Philadelphia, PA, USA

Aynharan Sinnarajah, MD, MPH
Division of Palliative Medicine
Department of Oncology
Cumming School of Medicine
University of Calgary
Calgary, Alberta, Canada

Jacob J. Strand, MD
Department of General Internal Medicine
Section of Palliative Medicine
Mayo Clinic
Rochester, MN, USA

Breana L. Taylor, MD
Department of Neurology
University of Washington
Seattle, WA, USA

Tobias Walbert, MD, PhD, MPH
Departments of Neurology and Neurosurgery
Henry Ford Health System
Detroit, MI, USA

Ludo J. Vanopdenbosch, MD
Department of Neurology
AZ Sint Jan Brugge Oostende
Bruges, Belgium

Palliative medicine is specialized care for patients and their families who are facing serious or advanced medical conditions [1], and it can be offered to patients at any stage of their illness, even at the time of diagnosis [2, 3]. A palliative approach to care can be provided in tandem with curative or disease-directed therapies [4–6]. The provision of palliative care may be by a patient's primary care physician, neurologist, geriatrician, other care provider, or a palliative care clinician.

Palliative care interventions focus on recognizing, preventing, and alleviating suffering [7] through effective symptom management, goals-of-care conversations, support for patients and caregivers, and advance care planning. There are eight recognized domains of palliative care – Structure and Process of Care, Physical Aspects of Care, Psychological Aspects of Care, Social Aspects of Care, Spiritual Aspects of Care, Cultural Aspects of Care, Care of the Patient at the End of Life, and Ethical and Legal Aspects of Care – which collectively evaluate a person's physical, psychological, spiritual, and social circumstances [8].

1. Structure and process of care explores a person's understanding of the disease process and the role of palliative care in their care plan. The palliative interdisciplinary team, which may consist of physicians, nurses, social workers, chaplains, pharmacists, and therapists, is highlighted.
2. Physical aspects of care relates to the management of physical symptoms through pharmacologic and non-pharmacologic approaches.
3. Psychological aspects of care focuses on the psychiatric and psychological needs of patients, existential distress, coping for patients and family members, and bereavement support.
4. Social aspects of care refers to the family structure, and this domain explores how social support can be optimized to improve the quality of life for the patient and caregivers.
5. Spiritual aspects of care includes a spiritual assessment, which explores spiritual, religious,

and meaning-based practices employed by the patient.
6. Cultural aspects of care broadly encompasses a person's race, ethnicity, language, nationality, socioeconomic status, and sexuality, and the impact that these factors may have on their decision-making and understanding of their disease.
7. Care of the patient at the end of life addresses the needs of patients who are in the dying process and of their family members.
8. Ethical and legal aspects of care addresses the decision-making capacity of the patient, the identification of a health care surrogate, and the completion of documents such as an advance directive that identify the care the patient desires at the end of life.

Palliative interventions have demonstrated higher satisfaction among patients and caregivers, increased quality of life, and reduced symptom burden among patients [9]. Patients with neurologic diseases that are progressive and incurable can benefit from a palliative approach to care given the expected and realized physical and cognitive decline. Neuropalliative care is a burgeoning subspecialty that focuses on the palliative needs of patients with neurologic disease and their family [10–13].

Important Considerations at the Time of Diagnosis

- Discussion regarding the disease
  - What does this mean for the patient/family?
- Symptom management
- Mood and coping
  - Depression, anxiety, frustration
  - Situational mood disorders
  - Support system
- Progression of disease/disease trajectory
- Advance care planning

- – Health Care Surrogate
- – Living Will
- – Estate/Financial Planning

Suggested Reading

1. Center to Advance Palliative Care. *Center to Advance Palliative Care Definition of Palliative Care.* www.capc .org/about/palliative-care/. Accessed December 30, 2016.

2. Howie L, Peppercorn J. Early palliative care in cancer treatment: Rationale, evidence and clinical implications. *Therapeutic Advances in Medical Oncology.* 2013;5(6): 318–23.

3. Mitka M. Cancer experts recommend introducing palliative care at time of diagnosis. *JAMA.* 2012;307(12): 1241–2.

4. Holloway RG, Arnold RM, Creutzfeldt CJ, et al. Palliative and end-of-life care in stroke: A statement for healthcare professionals from the American Heart Association/American Stroke Association. *Stroke.* 2014;45(6):1887–1916.

5. Ferrell BR, Temel JS, Temin S, et al. Integration of palliative care into standard oncology care: American Society of Clinical Oncology clinical practice guideline update. *Journal of Clinical Oncology: Official Journal of the American Society of Clinical Oncology.* 2017;35 (1):96–112.

6. Potosek J, Curry M, Buss M, Chittenden E. Integration of palliative care in end-stage liver disease and liver transplantation. *Journal of Palliative Medicine.* 2014;17 (11):1271–7.

7. World Health Organization. *World Health Organization Definition of Palliative Care.* www.who .int/cancer/palliative/definition/en/. Accessed November 30, 2016.

8. National Consensus Project for Quality Palliative Care. *Clinical Practice Guidelines for Quality Palliative Care.* www.hpna.org/multimedia/NCP_Clinical_Practice_G uidelines_3rd_Edition.pdf. Accessed June 4, 2017.

9. Kavalieratos D, Corbelli J, Zhang D, et al. Association between palliative care and patient and caregiver outcomes: A systematic review and meta-analysis. *JAMA.* 2016;316(20):2104–14.

10. Robinson MT, Barrett KM. Emerging subspecialties in neurology: Neuropalliative care. *Neurology.* 2014;82 (21):e180–2.

11. Creutzfeldt CJ, Robinson MT, Holloway RG. Neurologists as primary palliative care providers: Communication and practice approaches. *Neurology Clinical Practice.* 2016;6(1):40–8.

12. Dallara A, Tolchin DW. Emerging subspecialties in neurology: Palliative care. *Neurology.* 2014;82(7):640–2.

13. Boersma I, Miyasaki J, Kutner J, Kluger B. Palliative care and neurology: Time for a paradigm shift. *Neurology.* 2014;83(6):561–7.

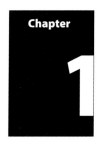

Chapter 1

The Role of Palliative Medicine in Neuropalliative Care

Daniel K. Partain and Jacob J. Strand

Clinical History

Mr. L is a 63-year-old gentleman from Wisconsin with systemic mastocytosis with associated clonal hematological non-mast cell lineage disease (SM-AHNMD), a rare hematologic illness. After unsuccessful treatment with six cycles of cladribine, the patient was enrolled in a clinical trial last month. He has been married to his wife for more than 30 years and maintains a very close relationship with his father and his dog. He is a Catholic and works as a long-haul truck driver. He loves fixing up old motorcycles, spending time with his dog, and dancing to blues music with his wife. After two weeks on the clinical trial, the patient experienced a large left hemispheric stroke with a completely occluded left internal carotid artery and left cavernous sinus thrombus. A left internal carotid artery thrombectomy was unsuccessful. The patient now has profound neurologic deficits including total left eye vision loss, non-fluent aphasia, and complete right hemiparesis/hemianesthesia. The patient is currently admitted to the neurologic intensive care unit (ICU) and his hematology physician is intimately involved with his care, making daily visits while in the ICU. Palliative medicine is consulted to assist with goals of care.

Introduction

Neurologic illnesses are often devastating and life-altering for patients, families, and medical teams. Not only do neurologic illnesses such as stroke, brain cancer, Parkinson disease, and multiple sclerosis have significant medical impacts across multiple domains of function such as gait, mobility, and eating but they also have profound impacts on nonmedical domains including self-identity and independence. The role of a palliative medicine physician includes elucidating the medical implications of neurologic illness and a patient's personal goals, preferences, and values, as well as developing an understanding of the complex interplay between the two. Although advance care planning can be done by anyone, it is a difficult task to do well, and it requires practice and training [1]. Thus, palliative medicine maintains an important role in assisting neurologic patients with clarifying the interactions between their personal values and the complexities of their current medical reality. In this chapter, we discuss the role of palliative medicine consultation in patients with neurologic illness.

The Role of a Palliative Care Consult

A palliative care consult in general can be divided into one of two requests: assistance with complex pain and symptom management or clarification of goals of care. While palliative medicine specialists receive specialized training on complex symptom management, this chapter focuses on the role of a palliative care consultant in communication between the patient/family and the medical team. The primary goal of a palliative care consultation is to provide the patient with goal-concordant care, or care that is aligned with their personal goals, preferences, and values.

A Understanding the Patient as a Whole Person

Effective communication about serious illness is a difficult challenge, but there is evidence that good communication improves patient and family satisfaction, improves hospice use, decreases aggressive end-of-life care, limits chemotherapy use in the last two weeks of life, and decreases depressive symptoms in both patients and their families. Patients want to know what to expect during the course of their illness, including how to plan for events that follow death. Indeed, patients fear a bad death much more than death itself [2]. Patients consistently rank nonmedical items as important in the course of serious illness, including preparation for death, achieving a sense of completion, decisions about treatment preferences, and being treated as a whole person [3].

Many proposed methods and models of communication regarding serious illness have emerged in the past two decades. One of the earliest discussions of the topic of physician–patient communication outlined four models of communication with a focus on the so-called deliberative model where physicians help patients to choose the best choice for them based on an exploration of their personal values while weighing the medical realities and available treatment options [4]. In the deliberative model of communication, the physician acts like a friend or teacher to help the patient make a decision. However, as can be seen in our patient scenario, many factors play into patient decision-making, and understanding the patient as a whole person is crucial in making recommendations for appropriate medical treatment.

B Discussing Nonmedical Topics with the Patient and Family

The beginning of an effective palliative care consultation is establishing rapport and learning about who the patient is as a person. We generally begin with open-ended questions and try to cover critical areas of a patient's life such as home environment, family relationships, spiritual/religious values, and level of function with activities of daily living. Many nonmedical issues are consistently rated as important by the majority of patients with serious illness, including cleanliness, being able to say goodbye to important people, resolving unfinished business, reviewing personal accomplishments, and maintaining one's dignity [3]. As such, a traditional medical interview would be unable to identify issues that are important to patients with serious illness. For example, in our patient scenario, simply asking questions about the patient's hematologic illness or neurologic deficits would not have allowed us to identify the most important people in his life, understand his family relationships, or become familiar with some of his personal accomplishments.

C Summarizing the Medical Situation

While most palliative medicine providers do not possess the expertise on pathophysiology, expected illness course, and treatment options for complex neurologic or neurosurgical diagnoses, they can provide value in a consultative role by communicating these things in a clear and concise manner to patients and families to allow them to make the most informed decision that would align with their goals, preferences, and values. Each palliative medicine provider has his or her own method and favored phrases, but a checklist approach that covers crucial conversation elements can be very helpful as an example of how to communicate a complex medical situation in simple terms. Preparation is the most important element before embarking on a discussion that summarizes a patient's medical situation and goals of care. Adequate preparation includes reviewing any previous advance directives on file and discussing the patient's medical situation with all relevant medical teams (in our scenario, relevant teams would be hematology and the neurology ICU teams) to get a sense of expected illness course, prognosis estimates, and treatment options. This preparation will allow for a meaningful discussion in which patients will have to make decisions based on this information.

A commonly used communication tool that highlights key elements of a goals of care discussion is the SPIKES communication tool. SPIKES is a mnemonic that stands for setting the scene, assessing the patient's perception, getting an invitation to discuss serious medical issues, providing knowledge, responding to concerns with empathy, and summarizing the conversation with a plan for what comes next [5].

D Discussing Prognosis

One of the most important roles of a palliative care physician during the consultation process is that of a prognosticator. Modern medicine has made tremendous advancements in diagnostic tools and new treatments, but providing an accurate prognosis still presents a unique and difficult challenge. In general, patients want to know what their illness is, how bad it is, and what can be done to treat it. Most physicians are able to reach a diagnosis and offer treatment options to patients, but the discussion of prognosis is often challenging. There are many barriers to discussing prognosis, including fear of death from the patient or the physician, discomfort with strong emotions, and concern about compromising the physician–patient relationship by eliminating hope.

Discussing prognosis has the potential to empower patients and allow them to make the best decisions about their health. Patients desire to know what to expect during the course of their illness, what may happen during the process of dying, and what

Table 1.1 The SPIKES protocol for breaking bad news

Communication Element	Examples
S – Setting the scene	Put pager and cell phone on silent/vibrate mode. Turn off patient television. Sit down. Say "There is some important information to share about your health; is everyone present that needs to be here?"
P – Patient perception	Ask "What do you understand about your illness?" Ask "What have the other doctors told you so far?"
I – Invitation to share	Ask "I have some information for you; is it okay if we talk about it together?"
K – Share knowledge	Discuss medical situation and prognosis in simple terms and in straightforward language.
E – Respond with empathy	Say "I can see that this is very difficult news for you." Say "This wasn't the news we were hoping for."
S – Summarize and plan for the future	Summarize the discussion in simple terms. Check in with the patient for understanding. Offer next steps, even if it is simply a return visit after the patient and family have had time to process difficult news.

happens after death. Patients also want to be able to review accomplishments, say goodbye, and achieve a sense of completion during the course of serious illness. In order to allow our patients to fulfill these needs and achieve a measure of self-actualization in the face of serious illness, prognosis must be discussed, and it should be done so gracefully.

Many physicians may find it difficult to discuss prognosis, but part of the process of a palliative care consultation is to know when it is most appropriate to have these conversations. By its very nature, a discussion of prognosis is a difficult conversation that involves significant emotional content from both the physician and the patient. Most patients in the United States prefer explicit information about their prognosis, but patients always maintain the right to dictate the content and flow of information and they may not always prefer explicit prognostic information. In general, it is appropriate to discuss prognosis in cases of imminent death, patient/family inquiries about hospice, or when discussing treatment options with a very low probability of success. A discussion of prognosis is also suggested when the physician would not be surprised if the patient died in the next 6–12 months [6].

E Negotiating Goals of Care

Understanding a patient's goals, preferences, and values is only part of the role of a palliative care consultation. The final part of a palliative care consult is the negotiation of a patient-centered plan in the context of the medical reality of serious illness. For example, most real-life medical scenarios have a very limited number of realistic treatment options, generally just two or three. In our patient with a large stroke, the realistic treatment options are limited to pursuing aggressive illness-directed therapy with a new clinical trial for his hematologic illness along with a comprehensive program of physical, occupational, and speech therapy or focusing on a comfort-directed approach to care with a focus on relief of bothersome symptoms and maximizing the patient's ability to function and accomplish his goals within a limited prognosis. However, just like anything else in medicine, the most patient-centered approach to care must be renegotiated on a regular basis as the clinical realities change. If a new experimental treatment is introduced that could potentially fit with a patient's goals of care, it is important to renegotiate the plan, as the patient's goals, preferences, and values are fluid and will change over time [7], particularly when their clinical status changes.

The process of negotiating goals of care involves many strong emotions, and several communication models are helpful in addressing situations in which strong emotions arise. A fundamental principle of addressing emotion is that patients are unable to process significant emotion and new facts at the

Table 1.2 The NURSE model, a tool for communicating emotions

Emotional Communication Tool	Examples
N – Name the emotion	"I can see that this makes you very sad." "I wonder if you might feel anger at this test result."
U – Understand the concern	"I can certainly understand why you'd be angry." "Many patients feel abandoned in this situation."
R – Respect the patient's effort	"I am very impressed at your positive attitude." "You have shown tremendous strength in a difficult time."
S – Support the patient	"I am here to walk with you during your suffering." "I will be your doctor until the end."
E – Explore complex emotions	"You seem angry and afraid; can you tell me more about how you're feeling?" "What do you mean when you say 'I can't believe this is happening after all I have done'?"

same time. When a patient is experiencing a strong emotion (e.g., sadness), it is more helpful to stop the conversation, acknowledge the emotion, respond with empathy, and allow the patient a chance to collect themselves before trying to impart new information. We are fond of the analogy of thinking of patients like a radio that can be tuned to either an emotional channel or a factual/rational channel, and they cannot play both channels at once. It is difficult to process new information until the loop is closed with a strong emotion. A frequently used communication tool for addressing emotion is the NURSE model. NURSE is a mnemonic that stands for naming, understanding, respecting, supporting, and exploring [8].

Conclusion

The process of doing a palliative care consult for a patient with serious neurologic illness offers many unique challenges, and thus we suggest consideration of a checklist approach to ensure that key elements of the consult are performed. One example of a comprehensive approach to a palliative care consult is the Serious Illness Communication Checklist, which integrates several communication models discussed earlier in this chapter [9]. The primary goal of a palliative care consult is to help the medical team provide goal-concordant care to the patient. Advance care planning and having difficult conversations that consider the patient as a whole person, understand nonmedical aspects of a patient's care, summarize the medical situation, discussing prognosis, and negotiating goals of care have been shown to improve the likelihood that patients' wishes are

followed (that is, improving the delivery of goal-concordant care) [10].

We now return to the case of Mr. L and put everything together to discuss the role of the palliative care consult in a patient with a serious neurologic illness. What follows is a discussion that took place with the patient and the final outcome. This discussion took place with several surrogate decision makers given that the patient's neurologic deficits did not allow for him to have decision-making capacity. His wife, Mrs. L, was his primary surrogate decision maker and was named in a health care proxy form.

PHYSICIAN: Good afternoon, Mrs. L. Can you tell me a little bit about your husband before he got sick?

MRS. L: He loved dancing to blues music, playing with his dog, and repairing motorcycles. He was very independent and didn't like anyone helping him. He hasn't really been to a doctor until he got this blood problem.

PHYSICIAN: It sounds like this process has been very hard for him. I'm hearing that his ability to use his hands was very important to him?

MRS. L: That's right. Not being able to work on his motorcycles or dance to his blues music is not what he would consider quality of life.

PHYSICIAN: I have some important information about your husband's health to share with you; are you ready to discuss this?

MRS. L: Yes, that is what we have been waiting for.

PHYSICIAN: The procedure that we tried to remove the blood clot from Mr. L's artery was not successful. Unfortunately, we do not think that his neurologic problems will get better, but instead might get worse. I do not think he would be able to fix motorcycles and dance to blues music again. We are worried that his neurologic condition may get worse, and he might die from this.

MRS. L: [Does not respond and begins to weep.]

PHYSICIAN: I can see that this is very upsetting news – it was not what we were hoping for. You have been so strong through this whole process, and this is a significant setback.

MRS. L: I knew this might happen, but I have so many emotions about this. I'm angry that the medicine for his blood problem didn't work. I'm sad that the blood clot removal wasn't successful. I'm worried about what might happen in the next few days.

PHYSICIAN: I can see why you would feel that way. I wish the medicine would have worked too.

MRS. L: What do we do next? Is he suffering?

PHYSICIAN: He does not seem to be experiencing any bothersome symptoms like pain right now. I think we should discuss whether we want to focus on Mr. L's illness by discussing other medications for his blood problem and aggressive physical therapy or focus on his quality of life by taking a more comfort-focused approach to his care.

MRS. L: I can't see that he would ever want to live this way with such a lack of mobility. I want to focus on his comfort.

The patient did not have any significant bothersome symptoms to address. We made arrangements for the patient to transition to hospice as soon as possible and discussed our conversation with the hematology team and the neurologic ICU team. Unfortunately, within the next three days, the patient became progressively unresponsive from brain herniation and died. We were at the bedside with the patient and his family and he died peacefully.

Suggested Reading

1. Tulsky JA, Chesney MA, Lo B. See one, do one, teach one? House staff experience discussing do-not-resuscitate orders. *Arch Intern Med.* 1996;**156**(12): 1285–9.

2. Steinhauser KE, Clipp EC, McNeilly M, Christakis NA, McIntyre LM, Tulsky JA. In search of a good death: Observations of patients, families, and providers. *Ann Intern Med.* 2000;**132**(10):825–32.

3. Steinhauser KE, Christakis NA, Clipp EC, McNeilly M, McIntyre L, Tulsky JA. Factors considered important at the end of life by patients, family, physicians, and other care providers. *JAMA.* 2000;**284**(19):2476–82.

4. Emanuel EJ, Emanuel LL. Four models of the physician–patient relationship. *JAMA.* 1992;**267**(16): 2221–6.

5. Baile WF, Buckman R, Lenzi R, Glober G, Beale EA, Kudelka AP. SPIKES – A six-step protocol for delivering bad news: Application to the patient with cancer. *Oncologist.* 2000;**5**(4):302–11.

6. Quill TE. Perspectives on care at the close of life. Initiating end-of-life discussions with seriously ill patients: Addressing the "elephant in the room." *JAMA.* 2000;**284**(19):2502–7.

7. Sudore RL, Fried TR. Redefining the "planning" in advance care planning: Preparing for end-of-life decision making. *Ann Intern Med.* 2010;**153**(4):256–61.

8. Pollak KI, Arnold RM, Jeffreys AS, Alexander SC, Olsen MK, Abernethy AP, et al. Oncologist communication about emotion during visits with patients with advanced cancer. *J Clin Oncol.* 2007;**25** (36):5748–52.

9. Bernacki RE, Block SD. Serious illness communications checklist. *Virtual Mentor.* 2013;**15** (12):1045–9.

10. Detering KM, Hancock AD, Reade MC, Silvester W. The impact of advance care planning on end of life care in elderly patients: Randomised controlled trial. *BMJ.* 2010;**340**:c1345.

Common Challenges in a Palliative Medicine Consultation

Daniel K. Partain and Jacob J. Strand

Clinical History

Mr. B is a 67-year-old gentleman from Minnesota who has been healthy for his entire life until having a seizure on Christmas Day of last year. He was eventually found to have glioblastoma multiforme (WHO grade IV), isocitrate dehydrogenase 1 (IDH-1) wild-type, methyl guanine methyl transferase (MGMT) non-methylated. He underwent resection followed by concurrent chemoradiation with temozolomide and 3,000 cGy of radiation. He continued adjuvant treatment with temozolomide and bevacizumab. He had recurrent disease approximately five months later and underwent another resection surgery.

Two months later, the patient was readmitted to the hospital with recurrent disease. The neurosurgical team took the patient to the operating room and discovered a highly invasive vascular tumor that was not amenable to resection. They were concerned that the patient would not be able to have another surgery and that his prognosis was quite poor. His hospital course was complicated by a surgical site infection and recurrent episodes of symptomatic supraventricular tachycardia requiring treatment with adenosine. Palliative medicine is consulted to discuss goals of care in a complex clinical situation.

Introduction

The role of a palliative medicine consultation in patients with serious neurologic and neurosurgical illnesses involves understanding the whole patient, discussing nonmedical issues with the patient, communicating prognosis, engaging in emotional conversations, and negotiating goals of care. Here, we discuss common challenges that may be encountered during a palliative medicine consultation and we suggest strategies on how to continue working with the patient and the medical team in the face of some of these challenges.

Common Challenges in Palliative Medicine Consultation

Palliative medicine is generally involved in the care of patients with serious or terminal illness, and thus it is a profession in which difficult conversations happen on a daily basis. Developing an understanding of some of the most common challenges is helpful in understanding the useful role that skilled palliative care clinicians can play for a patient with a serious neurologic illness. We present five common challenges, many of which will be encountered during the course of our patient case.

A Misunderstanding of Prognosis

Discussing prognosis gracefully in a way that can be easily understood by the patient and their family is a difficult skill. Any conversation where someone's life is discussed in terms of days, weeks, or months can be devastating and emotionally overwhelming. Physicians are often taught to communicate honestly while still preserving hope for a good outcome even in the face of very bad odds. As our medical technology evolves to push patients beyond previously established limits of human physiology, it is no surprise that a majority of patients feel that they can be cured from serious or terminal illnesses. Patients unfortunately do not understand their prognosis well. In one recent study, a third of patients with terminal cancer (stage IV small cell lung cancer) felt that their illness was totally curable, and almost three-quarters of patients felt that a reasonable goal of treatment was to get rid of all of their cancer [1].

The role of palliative care consultation involves clarification of prognosis and providing patients with relevant information to be able to make the most appropriate goal-concordant decisions about their health. It bears repeating that patients maintain the right to dictate the flow and content of information provided to them about their prognosis, but in general, patients prefer to know the most accurate information possible to have an opportunity to make appropriate plans and decisions about their care. Presenting a simple and clear message to a patient and their family with relevant prognostic information is an integral part of empowering a patient and providing them some control in the face of a serious illness that often strips them of their autonomy. Providing a consistent message across multiple conversations with the patient and their family increases the odds that a patient will gain an accurate understanding of their prognosis. It is also helpful to communicate the content of any prognostic discussions with the primary medical services so that all members of the medical team can maintain a consistent and clear estimate of prognosis.

B Strong Emotions That Impair Understanding and Judgment

People make decisions based on a number of factors, including facts, family, faith, fear, and many others. Only part of the decision-making process is based on factual information, as this information interacts with life experiences, worldview, and emotions to influence decisions. Thus, in the overwhelming experience of serious illness, it is understandable, or perhaps even expected, that strong emotions can influence decision-making. Physicians are taught to mix hope with reality, and indeed research has shown that patients want their doctors to discuss their illness with a mix of hope and explicit prognostic information [2]. Many physicians feel that their role is to continue to offer hope that their treatments will be curative.

As we saw earlier, simply asking patients if terminal cancer is curable or asking if chemotherapy can make all their cancer go away can influence almost a third of patients to change how they feel about their treatment options [1]. This is where a palliative medicine consult can be helpful. Most palliative medicine clinicians are not able to perform surgery, give radiation, or administer chemotherapy, and offering explicit prognostic information that is not directly tied to treatment options can help reduce the sense of presenting certain treatment options in a more positive light. Indeed, palliative medicine consultation significantly increases understanding of prognosis, and thus

increases the ability for patients to make appropriate decisions about their treatment [1].

C Concern about Discussing Sensitive Topics

Physicians may be uncomfortable addressing sensitive topics for a variety of reasons, including concern for compromising the physician–patient relationship, a feeling that they are unqualified to address nonmedical concerns, or concerns that they will eliminate the patient's hope by discussing difficult topics like death and dying. For example, many physicians feel that discussing religion and spirituality with their patients is more the responsibility of chaplain services, family members, or community leaders. In addition, they may feel unprepared to discuss topics outside of their comfort zone or in which they have no personal interest. However, while up to 87 percent of patients want some degree of religious/spiritual care from their physicians, 94 percent of patients with advanced terminal illness report no spiritual care from their physicians at all [3]. Moreover, despite the concern for eliminating hope, patients want their physicians to be comfortable talking about death and dying [4]. Palliative care physicians receive special training in these areas and can add significant value to the care of patients by discussing religion, spirituality, hope for miracles, death, dying, and the limits of medical science with patients in an open and candid manner to facilitate goal-concordant decision-making.

D Conflicting Goals, Preferences, and Values

All patients have goals, preferences, and values that interact within the context of their unique medical situation. Unfortunately, sometimes, patient goals come into conflict with the goals of the medical team or cannot be realistically accomplished in their particular medical reality. In addition, physicians are not good at predicting what patients want in a given situation, even if provided with a written advance directive [5]. Advance directive completion has increased significantly over the past two decades, but this has had relatively little impact on important patient outcomes such as death in the hospital [6]. Thus, while completion of an advance directive is certainly a good thing as it gets patients thinking about their health care and allows them to name a surrogate decision maker, it does not allow for patients to make decisions about the specific scenario they may face.

Palliative care consultation can be useful to help a patient understand their goals within the context of their particular illness and prognosis. A thorough discussion to gain insight into a patient's hopes, fears, trade-offs, and their own personal definition of quality of life can be very useful in providing appropriate care. One example of a framework to help clarify goals of care in a given scenario is the facilitated values history, which considers many domains of patient decision-making, including personal sense of well-being, maintenance of bodily integrity, maintenance of physical and cognitive function, autonomy/independence, social/emotional engagement, and adherence to spiritual beliefs [7].

Sometimes patient goals can conflict with what can realistically be accomplished or what the medical team can offer, and openly naming these realities and limitations can allow patients to make the best possible decisions. Mutually agreed-upon goals are one of the most important facilitators of good physician–patient communication; palliative medicine physicians can enable this process with clear information, empowering the patient to take an active role in making decisions, and being empathetic and supportive during the process [8]. One favored tool of creating alignment with patients and simultaneously expressing that their request is not possible is the wish/worry statement. When a patient says that they are certain the next line of chemotherapy will work, responding with a "wish/worry statement" (e.g., "I wish the chemotherapy would work that way") implies that their request is not possible, while aligning yourself with the patient that you share the same hope they do.

E Unrealistic or Impossible Patient/Family Expectations

Sometimes patients and their families will have unrealistic or impossible expectations despite multiple reasonable and thorough attempts to provide clear and concise information that what they are hoping for cannot be accomplished. For example, although almost three-quarters of patients with terminal cancer think their cancer can be eliminated with chemotherapy initially, only about 15 percent of patients remain unable to develop an accurate

assessment of their prognosis over time after involvement by a palliative care physician [1]. Even with persistent clear messages from a palliative medicine physician, some patients will not be able to accept or understand their illness for a variety of reasons, including strong emotions, poor medical insight, inability to remember key medical information, or religious beliefs. Patients who expect a miracle can be one of the most difficult challenges for a physician. A reasonable approach to patients who expect a miracle is to determine what a miracle means to that particular patient, provide a balanced and nonjudgmental response, and negotiate a patient-centered plan of care that honors their beliefs to the best of the ability of the medical team [9]. As with prognosis, communicating the content of these discussions to the rest of the medical team ensures a consistent message to maximize the likelihood that patients will gain an accurate understanding of their prognosis and what can reasonably be accomplished with regard to their treatment.

Conclusion

Palliative medicine consultation in serious neurologic illness can offer significant value to patients to relieve bothersome symptoms and clarify goals of care. However, there are many challenges, including strong emotions, religious/spiritual beliefs, concerns about discussing sensitive topics, difficulty communicating and understanding prognosis, and patients who expect a miracle despite a terminal illness. We have discussed some approaches and techniques to deal with these barriers to goal-concordant care. As with any difficult medical procedure, a goals-of-care discussion requires a systematic approach to have the best outcomes [10]. We conclude by returning to our case of Mr. B, a 67-year-old gentleman with recurrent glioblastoma multiforme.

PHYSICIAN: Hello, Mr. B. I am with the palliative medicine team. Can you tell me a little bit about yourself?

MR. B: Hey, Doc. Well, I am married with three children and I served in the Vietnam War.

PHYSICIAN: Thank you for your service to our country. Can you tell me what you understand about what's been going on with your health?

MR. B: Yeah, the surgeon said that I have a recurrent brain tumor and he's not sure if they can operate on me. I don't understand what happened – the other operations went just fine. Why can't they just operate on me again?

PHYSICIAN: It sounds like you're disappointed that the surgeon might not be able to take out your tumor, is that right?

MR. B: I mean, I guess I knew that eventually this might happen, I guess I just wasn't prepared to think about it.

PHYSICIAN: Can you tell me what you are most worried about?

MR. B: Well, I thought this thing was curable. The doctors always said I could get more surgery or have different chemotherapy. I don't know what happened.

PHYSICIAN: I want to share with you what I understand about your illness, are you ready to talk about that?

MR. B: No, I don't think so; I would like my wife to be here for anything like that. We made arrangements to come back later in the afternoon when the patient's wife would be present. It is always important to make sure that all key participants are available for meetings where goals, preferences, and values are discussed in significant detail. In the intervening hours, the patient developed some mild encephalopathy due to his surgical site infection that was complicated by encephalitis. He also had another episode of supraventricular tachycardia (SVT) that required treatment with adenosine. We discussed his care with the electrophysiology consultant on call. She offered an ablation procedure, but discussed that it would be very high risk and that the patient could die from a brain hemorrhage during or after the procedure.

PHYSICIAN: Hello, Mr. B. I'm afraid I have some difficult news to discuss, is now a good time?

MR. B: Yes, thank you for waiting for my wife.

PHYSICIAN: Unfortunately, the brain tumor has come back in such a way that we cannot do surgery. Since you have already had radiation to that area, we also cannot give you any more radiation. I am worried that time is shorter than what we are hoping for. Can you help me understand what is most important to you now?

MR. B: I don't understand what you mean. I was told that this is a curable problem. Can't I get more chemotherapy? I thought this place could perform miracles.

PHYSICIAN: I wish more chemotherapy would help, but I am worried that there are no more cancer-directed treatments that we can give. Can you tell me more about what you mean by a miracle?

MR. B: Well, I want to be cured. I don't want to leave my wife alone. Are you saying that my cancer is not curable?

PHYSICIAN: I'm afraid not. Your brain tumor, called a glioblastoma multiforme, or GBM for short, is a very aggressive brain tumor with a prognosis that is usually measured in months. Unfortunately, because of your infection and heart problem, I am concerned that time might be shorter than we were hoping for.

MR. B: Wow. That is very unexpected news. Well, I guess I need to know how long I've got so I can get things taken care of for my wife. Can you tell me how long I might have?

PHYSICIAN: I have discussed your care in detail with the neurosurgical doctors who know your illness the best. I think that you may have weeks to months given the aggressive nature of your tumor and your new infection.

MR. B: You know, if this can't be fixed, I think I want to go to hospice so I can spend time with my wife.

PHYSICIAN: That would be a very reasonable approach where we can focus on your comfort and quality of life.

MR. B: Well, what about this heart thing? I feel really terrible when my heart goes into that rhythm. Can you put a stop to that?

PHYSICIAN: We can do a special procedure where we burn a tiny portion of the heart muscle to stop that heart rhythm, but it's very high risk and you could potentially die from bleeding.

MR. B: I tell you what, I feel just terrible when these rhythms come on. I think I want to try for this procedure and then go to hospice. I can't enjoy my time outside the hospital if I'm constantly worrying about this heart problem.

Several barriers to goal-concordant care are shown in this case example, including unrealistic expectations, misunderstanding of prognosis, conflicting goals of care, and hoping for a miracle. Over the following days, it became apparent that the patient and his wife had previously had a fairly limited understanding of the nature of glioblastoma multiforme and had not been prepared to talk about death and dying before the current hospitalization. Ultimately, the patient decided to go for an ablation, a reasonable choice given his ongoing severe symptomatic SVT requiring frequent adenosine administration that would not have been available in hospice. He had several days in the hospital awaiting the ablation when he was able to spend time with his wife and daughter at the bedside discussing memories, saying goodbye, and getting important affairs in order. The patient ultimately died a few days after the ablation from a catastrophic brain hemorrhage. The last thing his wife shared with us is that he died without regrets, and the family was in complete agreement to accept the risks of the procedure to maximize his comfort outside the hospital.

Suggested Reading

1. Temel JS, Greer JA, Admane S, Gallagher ER, Jackson VA, Lynch TJ, et al. Longitudinal perceptions of prognosis and goals of therapy in patients with metastatic non-small-cell lung cancer: Results of a randomized study of early palliative care. *J Clin Oncol.* 2011;**29**(17):2319–26.

2. Curtis JR, Engelberg R, Young JP, Vig LK, Reinke LF, Wenrich MD, et al. An approach to understanding the interaction of hope and desire for explicit prognostic information among individuals with severe chronic obstructive pulmonary disease or advanced cancer. *J Palliat Med.* 2008;**11**(4): 610–20.

3. Balboni MJ, Sullivan A, Amobi A, Phelps AC, Gorman DP, Zollfrank A, et al. Why is spiritual care infrequent at the end of life? Spiritual care perceptions among patients, nurses, and physicians and the role of training. *J Clin Oncol.* 2013;**31**(4):461–7.

4. Steinhauser KE, Christakis NA, Clipp EC, McNeilly M, Grambow S, Parker J, et al. Preparing for the end of life: Preferences of patients, families, physicians, and other care providers. *J Pain Symptom Manage.* 2001;**22**(3): 727–37.

5. Coppola KM, Ditto PH, Danks JH, Smucker WD. Accuracy of primary care and hospital-based physicians' predictions of elderly outpatients' treatment preferences with and without advance directives. *Arch Intern Med.* 2001;**161**(3):431–40.

6. Silveira MJ, Wiitala W, Piette J. Advance directive completion by elderly Americans: A decade of change. *J Am Geriatr Soc.* 2014;**62**(4):706–10.

7. Scheunemann LP, Arnold RM, White DB. The facilitated values history: Helping surrogates make authentic decisions for incapacitated patients with advanced illness. *Am J Respir Crit Care Med.* 2012;**186** (6):480–6.

8. Stewart M, Brown JB, Boon H, Galajda J, Meredith L, Sangster M. Evidence on patient–doctor communication. *Cancer Prev Control.* 1999;**3**(1):25–30.

9. Delisser HM. A practical approach to the family that expects a miracle. *Chest.* 2009;**135**(6):1643–7.

10. Bernacki RE, Block SD, American College of Physicians High Value Care Task Force. Communication about serious illness care goals: A review and synthesis of best practices. *JAMA Intern Med.* 2014;**174**(12):1994–2003.

When Is the Right Time to Give Up?

William P. Cheshire Jr.

Clinical History

A 66-year-old man with a history of untreated hypertension presented to the emergency department with the sudden onset of headache and neck and bilateral shoulder pain. Upon evaluation, his blood pressure was 225/150 mmHg. Head CT demonstrated acute subarachnoid hemorrhage throughout the basilar cisterns (Figure 3.1). Cerebral arteriography located the source of hemorrhage, which was a spinal dural arteriovenous fistula arising from a radiculomeningeal feeder of the right vertebral artery at the C3 level. Attempted embolization was unsuccessful, with loss of motor-evoked potentials during the procedure.

Over the next five days, he became progressively quadriplegic, losing nearly all voluntary limb movement as well as voluntary respiration. MRI disclosed extensive brain stem and cervical spinal cord ischemia with cord edema (Figure 3.2), which was treated with dexamethasone and surgical decompression, but without improvement in neurologic status. He also received nimodipine for vasospasm, labetalol and hydralazine for blood pressure control, and oxycodone for headache.

Three days after the onset of quadriplegia and five days into his illness, his neurologic status had not changed further. When, on morning rounds, his

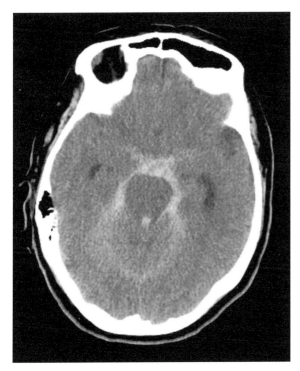

Figure 3.1 Axial CT of the brain demonstrating diffuse high density throughout the basal cisterns consistent with acute subarachnoid hemorrhage

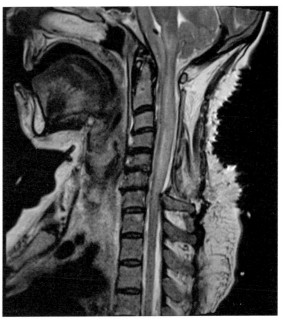

Figure 3.2 Sagittal FLAIR MRI of the cervical spine. There is increased signal intensity consistent with ischemic change within the central portion of the cervical cord from the level of the dens to C5 as well as within the medulla oblongata. Residual blood products are present ventral to the cord. Posterior elements of the cervical spine are absent, consistent with recent surgical decompression of the spinal cord.

physician asked how he was doing, he mouthed the words, "let me go."

Examination

The patient was alert and coherent, following commands, had a tracheostomy, and was mechanically ventilated. In addition to right facial weakness, left abducens palsy, and upper extremity hyporeflexia, minimal voluntary movement of any of his limbs could be elicited.

Palliative Domain of Care

Ethical and Legal Aspects of Care

Although the patient had not completed an advance directive, he retained decision-making capacity. Further discussion with the patient and his family clarified that the patient felt that he would not want to be kept alive in his current state of disability. His family members were in agreement with his wishes to withdraw life-sustaining treatments.

In regard to recommendations for proceeding with or withdrawing interventions, his care team was divided. Accepting the devastating impact of his neurologic injuries, one group empathized with the patient in his discouragement, as he faced the prospect of spending the remainder of his days unable to walk, transfer himself, use his hands, feed himself, attend to ordinary hygiene, or breathe on his own. Being ever more bedbound, totally dependent on others for basic care, constantly connected to a ventilator, having an indwelling catheter, being subject to skin breakdown, and experiencing profound loss of independence seemed intolerably burdensome. Furthermore, whether he had adequate insurance to cover the ongoing cost of skilled nursing care was uncertain, and the potential financial expense to his family might be considerable. Respecting the patient's autonomy seemed the right thing to do. The question remained, when was the right time to withdraw life-sustaining treatment?

The other group paused to consider that it was too early in the course of his illness to know his neurologic prognosis with certainty. Less than a week had passed, and they held out hope that some of his neurologic deficits might recover over the next few weeks as the vasospasm and edema resolved. The medical and surgical teams had worked diligently around the clock to provide the very best of care and the most advanced technology to give the patient the greatest possible chance to survive and to recover a meaningful quality of life. They had given of their skills and effort and felt personally invested in his care. They believed there was still a possibility for improvement and were not ready to give up. He was, after all, cognitively intact. It would be difficult to let die someone who was conscious, communicating, and through the experience of acute illness had formed a relationship with members of his care team. They felt that, as they had cared for him during the intense events of his hospitalization, they had gotten to know him. If they were to relinquish treatment this soon, even at his request, they might feel that they had failed to see him through his illness.

The team did not hesitate to honor the patient's wish to transition from full code to "do not resuscitate" (DNR) status, but could not agree whether to withdraw life-sustaining therapy at that time and called for ethics and palliative care consultations.

Palliative Care Discussion

The ethics committee affirmed the fundamental ethical principle that the patient, as an adult with the capacity to make decisions, has the ethical and legal right to forgo medical treatment, even life-sustaining interventions such as mechanical ventilation. However, this exercise of autonomy presupposes that the patient is informed. Truly informed consent requires several conditions to be met. There must be adequate disclosure of the information necessary to allow a reasonable person to make a prudent treatment choice. The patient must be able to comprehend the information and possess the cognitive capacity to make a decision. The patient must be free from coercion and give consent that is voluntary.

The neurologic consequences of a high-level spinal cord injury are complex. The discussion with the patient included information about what it means to have loss of voluntary arm and leg movement, loss of mobility, muscle atrophy, spasticity, limb contractures, loss of limb sensation, loss of bowel and bladder control, loss of sexual function, autonomic dysreflexia, and, at the C3 level, loss of voluntary respiration. Receiving this information is emotionally overwhelming, even for a cognitively intact patient, and takes time to assimilate. Adequate disclosure also includes information about the full range of rehabilitation options, and not only in the abstract, as knowledge of what is possible through rehabilitation is also experiential. It is impossible fully to know what it is like to live as a quadriplegic unless one experiences that life.

Not only is this information overwhelming, it is also frightening. This patient, who, prior to his illness, had worked as a baker, faced the prospect of loss of income. The ethics committee was concerned that his desire to have life-sustaining treatment withdrawn might have been influenced by his worries about whether he would have the financial means to pay his medical bills or whether his insurance would cover rehabilitation and long-term care – information not yet available just five days into his hospitalization. Another concern was social support. As a widower, he lived alone and faced the prospect of spending his remaining days in a nursing home, unless his daughter was willing to move cross-country and live with him – a question that would take time to resolve. The patient's family shared that he had always been an independent and self-sufficient person and that now he was forced to come to terms with the prospect of losing his independence. Was his wish to withdraw life-sustaining treatment a final expression of his self-determining personality trait? The ethics committee also learned that he had a history of depression. It was difficult to determine whether his spirit of resignation now might be a sign of recurrent depression. All of these factors were themselves coercive and, in the judgment of the ethics committee, could potentially impinge on his capacity to reach a decision now that, when in the future he were to look back on it, he would believe was the right decision for him.

The ethics committee noted the precedent that there have been cases with high-level cervical spinal cord injuries that were granted permission by the courts to discontinue life-sustaining treatment. In those cases the patients were beyond the acute phase of their injuries when they reached their decisions. The ethics committee advised the critical care team to defer a decision while giving the patient time to process this avalanche of new information and for the medical prognosis and rehabilitation options to become clearer.

The palliative care consultant clarified the goals of care and addressed further issues that contributed to the patient's weariness and that may have influenced the patient's desire to forego life support. The first was pain. His headache, which was no longer responding to treatment, came under control when oxycodone was switched to fentanyl. However, the increased amount of opioid medication had caused nausea and constipation. Following an enema and a regimen of milk of magnesia and ondansetron, the patient appeared more relaxed. A small dose of lorazepam at bedtime eased his anxiety and allowed him to obtain better sleep, and he began to appear more rested during the day. Pastoral care visited his bedside and provided spiritual support through prayer and scripture readings. His mood improved, and he began to ask more questions about rehabilitation possibilities.

Hospital Course

The patient's neurologic condition did not improve. The findings on his cervical spine MRI indicated a devastating injury with a poor prognosis and extremely limited rehabilitation potential.

The patient was given an opportunity to ask questions and to gain an understanding of his medical condition and the ways in which it would permanently impact his life. In conversation with his family and medical team, he was clear and persistent in articulating that he did not wish to continue life-sustaining treatment if there was no hope of recovery to an independent lifestyle or the ability to breathe on his own. The care team and palliative care consultant, in speaking with the patient, felt certain that the patient's decision was independent of his desire for pain control and not a manifestation of depression.

Ultimately, the patient was withdrawn from life-sustaining treatment, but not among the high-tech machines and beeping alarms and turmoil of the intensive care unit. The patient chose the option of discharge to hospice, where he was kept comfortable, his family by his side, until he felt ready to withdraw from the ventilator. During his last few days, as he slowly mouthed words to his son and daughter, he shared stories from his youth that they had never known, or perhaps had forgotten. His pet Sheltie was allowed to visit, and when she licked his hand, he smiled, even though he could feel nothing. A week later, while his family was at his bedside, he signaled that he was ready to go and asked to be disconnected from the ventilator. His son obliged. Then all was quiet.

General Remarks

This is an instance of, not one, but two sudden devastating neurologic injuries, a subarachnoid hemorrhage followed by a high-level cervical spinal cord injury, which left the patient permanently quadriplegic, immobile, and unable to breathe on his own. It is not unusual for patients with severe cervical spinal cord injuries, whether vascular or traumatic, to desire death acutely and yet, following rehabilitation, change their minds and choose to continue living. Long-term studies of spinal cord injury have shown that patients' perception of quality of life can improve over time. In this case, the patient chose not to be kept alive, and his care team appropriately honored his request, but not without first assessing and addressing the ethical and palliative factors relevant to that decision.

Whereas the patient's autonomy must be respected, including a decision to forego life-sustaining treatment, the patient must also be given adequate information to make an informed decision about treatment options. In the setting of an overwhelming injury, time is needed to acquire and process that information.

Meanwhile, there is much that palliative care can do to meet the patient's needs, clarify and address goals of care, and provide comfort. Palliative care is important for maximizing the dying patient's quality of life, including relieving the patient of burdensome symptoms that can make decisions regarding treatment more difficult.

Suggested Reading

Bracken MB, Shepard MJ, Webb SB, Jr. Psychological responses to acute spinal cord injury: An epidemiological study. *Paraplegia*. 1981;**19**:271–83.

Charlifue S, Apple D, Burns SP, et al. Mechanical ventilation, health, and quality of life following spinal cord injury. *Arch Phys Med Rehabil*. 2011;**92**:457–63.

Dijkers MPJM. Quality of life of individuals with spinal cord injury: A review of conceptualization, measurement, and research findings. *JRRD*. 2005;**42**:87–110.

Lemke DM. Patient-requested removal of ventilatory support in high-level tetraplegia: Guidelines for the health care provider. *SCI Nursing*. 2001;**18**:67–73.

Patterson DR, Miller-Perrin C, McCormick TR, Hudson LD. *N Engl J Med*. 1993;**328**:506–9.

Tada JE. *Joni: An Unforgettable Story*. Grand Rapids, MI: Zondervan, 2001.

Trevor-Deutsch B, Nelson RF. Refusal of treatment, leading to death: Towards optimization of informed consent. *Annals RCPSC*. 1996;**29**:487–9.

Volpe RL, Crites JS, Kirschner KL. Temporizing after spinal cord injury. *Hastings Cent Rep*. 2015;**45**:8–10.

Weller DJ, Miller PM. Emotional reactions of patient, family, and staff in acute-care period of spinal cord injury (parts 1 and 2). *Soc Work Health Care*. 1977;**2**:369–77, **3**:7–17.

A Request for Cognitive Enhancement

William P. Cheshire Jr.

Clinical History

A 24-year-old female law student presented to the neurology outpatient clinic one week following a minor head injury. She explained that her vehicle was rear-ended at low velocity, and although there was no head impact or loss of consciousness, she experienced some dizziness for a few days and still had an occipital headache, noise sensitivity, and "brain fog." MRI of the brain was reassuringly normal (Figure 4.1). The neurologist diagnosed post-traumatic headache and prescribed amitriptyline 25 mg at bedtime. She returned a month later to report that the headache had resolved. She discontinued the amitriptyline and was able to return to all of her usual activities.

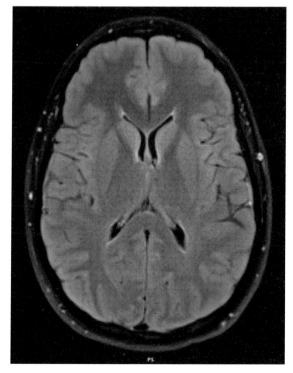

Figure 4.1 Normal axial FLAIR MRI of the brain

A short time later she visited her brother-in-law, who carries a diagnosis of attention deficit hyperactivity disorder (ADHD), for which he takes prescription amphetamine salts (brand name Adderall). She mentioned to him that, ever since the concussion, her mental concentration had been diminished. At times she struggled to keep up with her legal studies, and while she did complete her assignments on time, it required effort. When writing papers or reviewing notes, her thoughts tended to wander, and her mind did not consistently remain on task. He responded that her symptoms sounded a lot like his own, and so he offered her a few of his pills of amphetamine salts to try. She clearly does not meet diagnostic criteria for ADHD herself, but she tried the pills and felt that they transiently improved her concentration.

A year later, all of her post-concussive symptoms have fully resolved. She has no headache or brain fog and takes no medication. Her grades and other indicators of academic performance have returned to her usual level. In fact, her standing is in the top 10 percent of her class. She is an ambitious student and, upon graduation, she aspires to join the most prestigious law firm in her city. The competition for the entry-level position is fierce, and to succeed, she believes that she must excel enough to reach the top 5 percent of her class. When she pushes herself even harder, studying through the night and cutting short her sleep, she later feels constrained by fatigue. She feels that she needs a further edge.

She returns to the neurologist to request a prescription for amphetamine salts to enable her to improve her academic performance beyond her normal capacity. As final exams are approaching, she inquires whether it would be possible to obtain a prescription for a dose higher than what her brother-in-law takes.

Examination

The patient is alert, intelligent, and coherent, though somewhat anxious. Neurologic examination, including mental status, is normal.

Palliative Domains of Care

Ethical and Legal Aspects of Care, Physical and Psychological Aspects of Care

Among the range of problems addressed by palliative medicine are headache, cognitive impairment, dizziness, and fatigue, all of which can present with vague symptoms in the absence of objective deficits or imaging abnormalities, and yet for the patient they can be quite disabling. For each of these problems, the goal of care is improvement in symptoms and restoration of function and quality of life.

When the patient's goals of care go beyond therapy to the application of medical treatment for the purpose of surpassing the functional capacity she has in health, perhaps to achieve a state of superhealth, then the desire is no longer for palliation but for enhancement. Historically, physicians have understood the proper role of medicine to be the treatment and prevention of disease and not the effort to make healthy persons better than well.

The boundary between therapy and enhancement can be ambiguous, and the approach to brain fog can be obscured by ethical fog. The ethical distinction between therapy and enhancement may not be apparent, for example, to the patient who has redefined her sense of personal identity as something greater than she now is, such that normal health to her now seems inadequate and perhaps in need of a medical solution. Moreover, the biological distinction between health and disease in this case may be unknowable to the physician, who may reasonably question whether some subtle effects of the mild concussion could persist due to diffuse axonal shearing or post-concussive neurochemical changes in the brain undetectable by MRI. Not just one but both treatment goals – enhancement and therapy – may apply, depending on how one interprets the ambiguous elements of this case.

Outpatient Course

The neurologist considered the patient's request in a nonjudgmental, empathetic manner, but declined to prescribe amphetamine salts, which are a controlled substance and not medically indicated or approved for the purpose of enhancing cognition. The neurologist's conclusion was also based on studies that have shown minimal improvement in objective measures of cognitive performance in subjects taking amphetamine salts as compared to placebo, although the subjects had the perception of enhanced performance. The neurologist also educated the patient about the health risks of taking amphetamine salts. They and other central nervous system stimulants frequently cause adverse effects that can include anxiety, insomnia, palpitations, and headache.

The neurologist probed further into the patient's lifestyle and discovered a number of remediable factors relevant to cognitive and academic performance. The patient had developed a habit of procrastinating until, the night before an assignment was due, she would drink coffee or highly caffeinated energy drinks to stay awake through the night to complete the work on time. The disruption in her sleep schedule rendered her fatigued for the next several days, causing her to slip further behind in her work. She attempted to combat her fatigue with high-calorie snacks rather than a balanced, nutritious diet. Because she felt fatigued, she was no longer exercising regularly. The combined effect was a vicious cycle of brief stimulation alternating with prolonged fatigue. Additionally, when studying, every few minutes she would glance at the latest e-mail alert or social media post appearing on her computer display. She believed these distractions were supplying the social connectedness that she did not otherwise have time for, but they also disrupted her train of thought. The important questions in her field of study and the complex answers to them no longer seemed to fit within her shrinking attention span.

Palliative Care Discussion

Palliation need not be pharmacologic. There were clearly a number of healthier opportunities in this case to improve the patient's energy level, academic performance, and sense of well-being without resorting to medication.

Mixed amphetamine salts and other psychostimulants, such as methylphenidate and modafinil, are widely used in the United States, sometimes as diverted prescriptions, by healthy students with the intent of cognitive enhancement. These drugs have but a small effect on cognition as compared to their perceived enhancement of performance. Furthermore, their users may underestimate the drugs' potential medical risks. Research is under way to develop more potent drugs to augment cognitive performance. Once such drugs are introduced for treatment of cognitive disorders, such as dementia, the option of using them off-label for enhancement of cognitive performance in healthy persons becomes available.

Proponents of cognitive enhancement of the healthy have argued that physicians should agree to prescribe such drugs for informed patients because it respects their autonomy. In respecting the patient's autonomy, it is necessary to distinguish between autonomy as a negative right versus autonomy as a positive right. Whereas the patient has an inviolable ethical and legal right to refuse any recommended medical intervention, it does not follow that the patient has a positive right to receive any medical intervention that is not recommended. Respect for autonomy is a fundamental principle of medical ethics, but it is not the only principle. Autonomy must be held in balance with other valid principles, including the principle of non-maleficence, which obligates the physician, in keeping with the Hippocratic tradition, "First, do no harm."

The argument from autonomy is undermined by the reality that a request for pharmacologic enhancement may not be fully autonomous. If one's competitors are availing themselves of an enhancement edge, a student or professional may feel at risk of falling behind by not utilizing the same advantage. Peer, academic, and professional competitive pressures can be compelling.

A further concern is that the attempt to alleviate perceived cognitive inadequacy by stimulant medication could place the ambitious student on an unsustainable performance trajectory. If medication were to enable her to stay awake longer and read more articles in an evening or score a few points higher on the next examination, she may adjust to this augmented level of performance as a "new normal" and set her future expectations accordingly. She would thus be dependent on ongoing use of the medication to maintain her new level of accomplishment. It might be difficult not to place undue emphasis on performance as an end in itself and to the neglect of other aspects of life. It might be difficult to resist taking even more of the drug in an attempt to push one's performance even higher.

For how long would a patient seeking enhancement remain on a stimulant drug? If the drug eventually had to be stopped because of adverse cardiac or psychological effects, the return to one's natural performance capacity might be experienced as failure.

General Remarks

Cerebral concussion is a common syndrome defined as "a clinical syndrome characterized by immediate and transient impairment of neural function, such as alteration of consciousness, disturbance of vision, equilibrium, etc., due to mechanical forces." Concussions can be difficult to diagnose because, in most cases, pathological changes cannot be visualized by neuroimaging. The head need not have struck an object. Rotational acceleration and deceleration generate destructive shear forces within the brain. Symptoms from mild concussions are typically most pronounced during the first day or two following injury and, in the majority of patients, resolve over days to weeks. Some will experience continued symptoms of post-concussion syndrome, which may include headache, dizziness, fatigue, irritability, anxiety, insomnia, or loss of mental concentration.

No scientifically established treatments are available for treating post-concussion syndrome. Limited data are available regarding pharmacologic treatment for cognitive symptoms. Whereas preliminary studies have reported improvement with donepezil or selective serotonin reuptake inhibitors (SSRIs) in some patients, a reasonable approach is to individualize treatment to the particular symptoms of each patient. Medications that are helpful in treating migraine and tension-type headache, for example, are appropriate in treating post-concussion headache. Insomnia is best managed initially with attention to good sleep hygiene. For anxiety or depression, anxiolytic or antidepressant medications may be appropriate. Patients who have had a concussion should be advised to avoid situations that place them at risk for a second concussion. Reassurance is also appropriate, as most patients will improve over a number of months.

Suggested Reading

Cheshire WP. Drugs for enhancing cognition and their ethical implications: A hot new cup of tea. *Expert Rev Neurother*. 2006;**6**:263–366.

Cheshire WP. The pharmacologically enhanced physician. *AMA J Ethics*. 2008;**10**:594–8.

Cheshire WP. Requests for enhanced function in healthy individuals. In Williams MA, McGuire D, Rizzo M, editors, *Practical Ethics in Clinical Neurology*.

Philadelphia, PA: Wolters Kluwer, Lippincott, Williams & Wilkins, 2012, pp. 190–202.

Congress of Neurological Surgeons. Committee on head injury nomenclature: Glossary of head injury. *Clin Neurosurg.* 1966;**12**:386–94.

Greely H, Sahakian B, Harris J, et al. Towards responsible use of cognitive-enhancing drugs by the healthy. *Nature.* 2008;**456**:702–5.

Ilieva I, Boland J, Farah MJ. Objective and subjective cognitive enhancing effects of mixed amphetamine salts in healthy people. *Neuropharmacology.* 2013;**64**:496–505.

Kass L. A Report of the President's Council on Bioethics. *Beyond Therapy: Biotechnology and the Pursuit of Happiness.* Washington, DC: Harper Perennial, 2003.

Meaney DF, Smith DH. Biomechanics of concussion. *Clin Sports Med.* 2011;**30**:19–31.

Ragan CI, Bard I, Singh I, Independent Scientific Committee on Drugs: What should we do about student use of cognitive enhancers? An analysis of current evidence. *Neuropharmacology.* 2013;**64**:588–95.

Weiss HD, Stern BJ, Goldberg J. Post-traumatic migraine: Chronic migraine precipitated by minor head or neck trauma. *Headache.* 1991;**31**:451–6.

"Doctor, How Long Does He Have?"

Paul Glare

Clinical History

A 58-year-old man with an 18-month history of glioblastoma multiforme suffers from headaches, memory loss, and personality changes. On this occasion, he presented to the emergency room (ER) with a two-day history of a worsening headache, a four-hour history of acute paresis of the right arm, and vertigo.

Examination

Alert, Glasgow Coma Score 15; vital signs were stable. He has an expressive aphasia and there is weakness and hyporeflexia of the right upper extremity. Plantar responses are flexor.

MRI of his brain showed recurrent, multifocal disease up to 2 cm in diameter with associated edema. IV dexamethasone (4 mg four times a day) is commenced. He is reviewed by the neurosurgery team and surgical intervention is not recommended. He is admitted to the floor and the neuro-oncology team reviews his case and recommends no further treatment, and a palliative care consult. The first thing his wife asks after you introduce yourself is, "Doctor, how long does he have?"

Palliative Domain of Care

Structure and Process of Care: Prognostication

One of the key roles for palliative care practitioners is to initiate discussions on prognosis and goals of care, which have often been neglected prior to the consultation occurring. Such discussions are the most common function performed by palliative care services, occurring in almost 95 percent of consults in one survey.

Predicting the time until death has always been an important role of the physician, dating back to Hippocrates. But formal medical education in this type of forecasting is now scarce. Consequently, "Doctor, how long do I have?" is one of the most intimidating questions asked of physicians. This may

be even more so when the question relates to a patient with a brain tumor, where patient responses to treatment are very variable, even for patients with the same tumor type.

Glioblastoma multiforme (GBM) is the commonest malignant primary brain tumor. With multimodal treatment, GBM has a median survival of approximately 15 months, but few patients survive longer than three years [1]. Historically, GBM patients have a better outlook if they are younger, experience seizures or cranial neuropathies, have encapsulated tumors, undergo resection (versus intraoperative biopsy only), or receive adjuvant chemotherapy and radiation therapy [2]. More recently, great progress has been made in identifying a range of biomarkers, molecular signatures and imaging modalities that predict gliomagenesis, tumor aggressiveness, and disease progression [3]. While they raise the hope of more effective personalized therapy, this kind of predictive factor does not help answer this patient's question. In patients with advanced disease, factors other than tumor-related ones are important for prognostication. They include performance status, symptoms, psychosocial factors, and abnormal lab values [4].

Palliative Care Discussion

In the days of yore, when diagnoses were inaccurate and effective treatments were lacking, expertise in prognostication was the predominant clinical skill indicating the physician's knowledge and mastery of disease. Thankfully, this kind of prognostication diminished during the twentieth century with the development of accurate diagnostic tests and effective therapies for many previously untreatable conditions. Prognostication has seen a resurgence in the era of hospice and palliative care as patients with progressive, eventually fatal illnesses such as GBM, and their families, seek information about their life expectancy to help plan realistically for their futures [5].

Due to the lapse in prognostication in the twentieth century, it is no longer part of the medical education curriculum, despite the fact that it is a frequently performed clinical act. Consequently, contemporary physicians find prognostication difficult and stressful. They prefer to avoid prognosticating, generally waiting to be asked rather than volunteering a prediction, especially when the clinical situation is atypical or the course seems more uncertain than usual. Physicians may also be less willing to prognosticate if they see prognostications as self-fulfilling prophecies that take away hope.

As a result, discussions about prognosis at the end of life often do not take place, and if they do, they are limited in scope. One chart review of advance care planning in inoperable cancer patients found discussions of prognosis were documented in only 38 percent of charts. Physicians and patients were both present during the discussion in 52 percent of them. Time until expected death was infrequently documented. At most, a physician may write a prognosis as "guarded," "poor," or "terminal," as if the profession had mutually agreed-upon objective definitions.

Because clarifying the prognosis is one of the key functions of hospital palliative care teams, their education and training needs to focus on overcoming these tendencies of avoidance and deception in the effort to provide a false hope. In the face of these norms, it's important to deconstruct the process of prognostication into its components and develop expertise in each:

- Formulating the prognosis
- Communicating it to the patient, family, or other professionals
- Using the prognosis appropriately and effectively

A Formulating the Prognosis

This can be done in two ways: by making (1) an objective prediction based on one or more established predictive factors, often combined in a mathematical model to provide a prognostic score or index; or (2) a subjective judgment, relying on past experience of other patients with similar problems. Objective prognostication based on established predictive factors has been called actuarial judgment, and clinical judgment formulated in one's head is called subjective judgment. Subjective judgment may be quasi-objective by taking into account things like the disease's trajectory, comorbidities, and beliefs about fighting spirit/ will to live.

Actuarial judgment is preferred over subjective judgment in most areas of health care, e.g., when diagnosing depression, but is problematic in predicting survival at the end of life, especially in this patient's case:

- Disease-specific prognostic tools have been developed for many cancers, but none exist for brain tumors.
- Prognostic tools have been developed for palliative care populations, but most excluded brain tumor patients from the study population.
- Some of the data to inputs (e.g., recent laboratory test results) may not be available.
- The tool's output may not provide prognostic information in a format that is relevant to the clinical situation.
- The predictions may be accurate for groups, but not at the individual level.

Because of these limitations, subjective judgment of survival remains an important competency for palliative care physicians if for no other reason than some of the actuarial tools include the subjective judgment as one of the inputs. In fact, a systematic review of clinicians' predictions of survival (CPS) in terminal cancer patients found that it accounted for approximately half of the variance in observed survival, greater than that explained by the more "objective" factors used in actuarial prognostic indices, such as performance status, symptoms, and abnormal lab values [6]. There was a positive linear correlation between predicted survival and actual survival to six months but not beyond, thus confirming physicians' ability to discriminate between groups of terminally ill cancer patients, according to their short-term survival. However, physicians are not well calibrated, as demonstrated by CPS being consistently inaccurate and biased in the overly optimistic direction – by as much as a factor of three to five. The experience and specialty of the physician and the nature of the physician–patient relationship may be confounders for the accuracy of the CPS. A prospective study of CPS when making referrals to a US hospice indicated academic oncologists were more accurate than community oncologists or family physicians and more experienced physicians were more accurate. However, this increased accuracy was blunted if the relationship between the physician and patient was strong [7]. This led the authors to suggest an experienced but dispassionate specialist physician was likely to be the most accurate and might be requested for a prognostic "second opinion" if an accurate prognosis was deemed essential (e.g., deciding to withdraw life-sustaining treatment).

A special kind of subjective judgment of prognosis is the so-called surprise question (SQ): "Would I be surprised if this patient died in (the time period of interest)?" The SQ has been shown to have a very high negative predictive value, with only 3 percent of "Yes, I would be surprised" patients dying, although it had only a modest positive predictive value [8]. It is being promoted in the British National Health Service's Gold Standards Framework as the cornerstone of determining hospice eligibility. Subjective prediction of survival is a valid means to obtain a general prognostic evaluation of patients, but is subject to a series of factors limiting its accuracy. Its use is recommended together with other prognostic factors.

At the very end of life, prognostication is synonymous with "diagnosing dying." The Palliative Performance Score (PPS) is a variation on the Karnofsky Performance Scale that uses ambulatory status, activities of daily living (ADLs), oral intake, and level of consciousness for scoring it. In the original study, patients with the lowest scores (10 percent, 20 percent, and 30 percent) had average survivals of two, three, and seven days, respectively [9]. Despite what many residents and nurses believe, clinicians and families cannot rely on changes in vital signs alone to rule in or rule out impending death. While associated with increased heart rate, decreased blood pressure (systolic and diastolic), and decreased oxygen saturation, these changes had high specificity (≥ 80 percent), low sensitivity (≤ 35 percent), and only modest positive likelihood ratios (≤ 5) for impending death within three days. A large proportion of patients have normal vital signs in the last days of life.

B Communication

Having formulated a prognosis, the physician needs to communicate this clearly but sensitively to the patient and family. There are many excellent articles on "how to break bad news" that describe how to go about this challenging task, of which disclosing a poor prognosis is often used as a teaching example. Some specific points regarding communicating prognosis are worth making to supplement the general communication skills literature.

- Most – but not all – patients and families want prognostic information; however, there are few studies to provide guidance on who wants it or what they want.
- It has been said patients and families both "dread and crave" prognostic information and want hopeful statements added with the less hopeful facts.
- Patients and families often want the physician to initiate prognostic discussions, but the norm for physicians is not to discuss it unless asked.
- There are large discrepancies between patients' and physicians' perceptions of how much prognostic information is wanted, given, and understood.
- Patient and family information needs vary across the course of the illness and they may want less as they enter the terminal phase of their illness.
- They also vary with age, race, and culture.
- They also vary in how they prefer the information presented (words, numbers, graphs), and by whom.

Survival predictions can be framed as "temporal" predictions, estimating the amount of time the person will live, expressed as a continuous variable (so many hours, days, weeks, or months), or else a categorical one (e.g., "hours to days," "days to weeks," "months to years"). Survival predictions can also be "probabilistic," expressing the percent chance of surviving to a certain time point (e.g., 50 percent chance of being alive in one month). Studies of CPS have tended to use temporal predictions, whereas most prognostic indexes provide probabilistic predictions. Therefore, presenting prognostic information involves numbers, time, and maybe probabilities, so a degree of numeracy is needed on the part of the patient/family – and the physician – for effective communication to occur. Temporal predictions ("he has six months to live") are easier to communicate than probabilistic ones, but are inaccurate except perhaps in the final month.

Even though "the median is not the message" and population-based median survivals (e.g., 15 months for GBM) are not very helpful for individual cases, knowing the median is useful when the shape of the Kaplan Meier survival curves for advanced cancers is taken into account [10]. Such curves typically follow an exponential function, so that 50 percent of individuals will die between the first and third quartiles, which tend to span from one half to double the median. Moreover, 80 percent (that is, all but the top and bottom decile) survive between one-sixth and four times the median (Figure 5.1), being from three

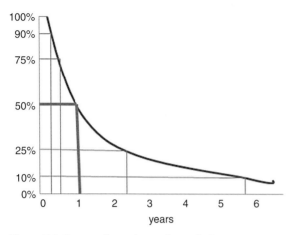

Figure 5.1 Cartoon of typical survival curve for brain tumor patients, indicating relationship between percentage survival and fractions/multiples of the median (bold lines)

months to six years for GBM. While this wide range seems to make prognostication farcical ("it could be as much as a few months or more than five years"), it is the basis for generating various statements that meet differing patients' needs and situations:

- "Patients with GBM typically live 15 months, give or take."
- "Half the patients with GBM live between eight months and two to three years."
- "I'd be surprised (< 10 percent chance) if you made five years."
- "I think you will probably (75 percent chance) make it to Thanksgiving this year but less likely (25 percent chance) for next year."

Even when prognosis is discussed, concerns remain about the openness of such discussions being "partial and conditional" rather than "full and open." Audiotaped consults have revealed a degree of collusion in physician–patient communication, driven by physicians' activism and patients' adherence to the treatment calendar and the "recovery plot," generating a "false optimism about recovery."

C Utilization

Disclosure of terminal prognosis is seen as ethically justified, especially in Western countries because it upholds the principle of self-determination and enables patients to make treatment decisions consistent with their life goals. Prognosis can be utilized in palliative care for various reasons, not just advance care planning:

- It is the legal basis for determining hospice eligibility.
- It is necessary for implementing and enforcing other palliative care laws, which some states now have.
- It is also the foundation for discussions on topics such as medical futility and palliative sedation, therefore it may be called into question in an ethics committee or a court of law.
- It is important in research, for study design and analysis.
- Most of all, it is a technical prerequisite for clinical decision-making in patients with eventually fatal illnesses.

An openly discussed prognosis has the potential to greatly alter the treatment plan for a patient. Patient-centered medical care depends on shared medical decision-making among the patient, family, and health care staff. To ensure adequate informed consent for ongoing care, the following areas should be reviewed as appropriate:

- a thorough appraisal of the clinical situation (diagnosis, comorbidities, pathology)
- the various treatment options based on the clinical situation
- the prognosis of the patient based on the possible treatments
- the preferences of informed patients or proxies

Without the inclusion of possible outcomes expected from a particular treatment course, informed consent and shared decision-making could be considered incomplete.

Clarification of prognosis is vital to ensure patients make decisions based on likely outcomes as opposed to merely hopeful results. One of the most robust modern studies on the impact of prognostication was the Study to Understand Prognoses and Preferences for Outcomes and Risks of Treatment (SUPPORT), in which prognostic information was explicitly provided to try to improve end-of-life care.

Using a computer-generated algorithm to prognosticate, SUPPORT demonstrated increased advance care planning discussions between patient and physician when the patient was given an objective estimate of prognosis of surviving two months of 40 percent or less. Other findings from SUPPORT included patients being less likely to desire cardiopulmonary resuscitation (CPR) if the patients felt the prognoses to be "poor." Other research has shown that knowledge of the statistics of CPR outcomes greatly decreased the likelihood of patients choosing CPR during an acute illness, and that watching a video depicting living with advanced dementia was associated with increased preference for comfort care over life-prolonging treatments by patients without dementia.

Multiple palliative care teams can attest to patients being optimistic in regards to prognosis in light of metastatic disease or incurable treatment options. This optimism of prognostication as perceived by patients may lead to the requesting of medical technologies and treatments that would not be chosen if a more accurate and realistic prognosis was formulated and clearly communicated. Palliative care teams frequently are able to realign goals of care based on prognostic information, and the landmark study of integrating palliative care with lung cancer treatment demonstrated that patients randomized to the palliative care arm received less aggressive care (33 percent versus 56 percent) at the end of life, and lived longer.

Prognostication can be used to assist decisions of patients and families about time shared together, estate management, funeral planning, and other practical issues. Prognosis is also important for families in determining how to respond to patients' palliative care needs, such as deciding how to care for the patients at home to urgently summoning a relative from out of town to visit a dying loved one. Parents of children with cancer who realize there is no hope of cure are also more likely to choose palliative care. The palliative care physician needs to be aware of these concerns when discussing prognosis and other end-of-life issues with families. Reviewing prognostic information repeatedly on multiple occasions is likely necessary to ensure adequate understanding by families.

Hospital Course

His condition stabilizes, but he remains totally bedbound and completely dependent in his ADLs. He is alert but having some difficulty swallowing and is allowed thickened fluids by the speech therapist. A disposition plan begins to be considered. How will this be formulated?

Discharge planning is a crucial function of palliative care consult services, with discharge plans being established for a majority of referrals. Predicting the outcome is one of many complex functions to be considered when developing a discharge plan in terminally ill patients, and often goes beyond "time-to-death" to include the other dimensions of prognosis. The typical palliative care consult, where decisions/goals are usually central, will involve predicting:

- the time frame of death
- the impact of disease-modifying therapies, including toxicities
- the future disease course (including symptoms, function, family impact, and financial issues)

The palliative care physician needs to integrate these prognostic data points into a cohesive whole and then match this information with the various options for providing the care (home, nursing home, hospice facility, hospital) and the patient and family's goals, priorities, and expectations. Will the patient become weaker or stronger? More or less mobile? Will the patient develop problems many families may have difficulty with (e.g., bleeding, incontinence, seizures, confusion)? Predicting these outcomes can be as difficult as predicting death.

After several family meetings, which included offering clarification that there are few remaining treatment options, especially in someone with such a poor performance status, they accept that the dying process has begun and they decide to forgo further disease specific measures and enroll in hospice. What needs to happen now?

In determining hospice eligibility, medical directors must specify that the individual's prognosis is for a life expectancy of six months or less if the terminal illness runs its normal course. Many hospices provide guidance to referring physicians on how to make a clinical determination of a six-month prognosis. For cancer patients, including brain tumors, these typically include:

- KPS or PPS < 70 percent
- Dependent in two of six ADLs
- Metastases at presentation **or** progression from an earlier stage of disease to metastatic disease with either
  - A continued decline in spite of therapy; or
  - Patient declines further directed therapy.

Certain cancers with poor prognoses (e.g., small cell lung, brain and pancreatic cancer) may be hospice eligible without fulfilling the other criteria.

The certifying physician must provide this clinical information and other documentation supporting the medical prognosis to accompany the certification and it must be filed in the medical record. The physician must include a brief narrative explanation of the clinical findings that support a life expectancy of six months or less and confirm that he/she composed the narrative based on his/her review of the patient's medical record or, if applicable, his/her examination of the patient.

General Remarks

Prognostication is an essential component of a palliative care consultation as it can influence patient and family goals and the focus of care. Clinicians should be able to effectively estimate the life expectancy for patients with serious illnesses, communicate the prognosis in an empathic manner to patients and families, and utilize the information appropriately to assist patients with developing a management plan.

Suggested Reading

1. Stupp R, Hegi ME, Mason WP, et al. Effects of radiotherapy with concomitant and adjuvant temozolomide versus radiotherapy alone on survival in glioblastoma in a randomised phase III study: 5-year analysis of the EORTC-NCIC trial. *Lancet Oncol.* 2009;**10**:459–66.

2. Gehan EA, Walker MD. Prognostic factors for patients with brain tumors. *Natl Cancer Inst Monogr.* 1977;**46**:189–95.

3. McNamara MG, Sahebjam S, Mason WP. Emerging biomarkers in glioblastoma. *Cancers (Basel).* 2013;**5**:1103–19.

4. Hauser CA, Stockler MR, Tattersall MH. Prognostic factors in patients with recently diagnosed incurable cancer: A systematic review. *Support Care Cancer.* 2006;**14**:999–1011.

5. Glare PA, Sinclair CT. Palliative medicine review: Prognostication. *J Palliat Med.* 2008;**11**:84–103.

6. Glare P, Virik K, Jones M, et al. A systematic review of physicians' survival predictions in terminally ill cancer patients. *BMJ.* 2003;**327**:195–8.

7. Christakis NA, Lamont EB. Extent and determinants of error in doctors' prognoses in terminally ill patients: Prospective cohort study. *BMJ.* 2000;**320**:469–72.

8. Moss AH, Lunney JR, Culp S, et al: Prognostic significance of the "surprise" question in cancer patients. *J Palliat Med.* 2010;**13**:837–40.

9. Anderson F, Downing GM, Hill J, et al. Palliative performance scale (PPS): A new tool. *J Palliat Care.* 1996;**12**:5–11.

10. Stockler MR, Tattersall MH, Boyer MJ, et al. Disarming the guarded prognosis: Predicting survival in newly referred patients with incurable cancer. *Br J Cancer.* 2006;**94**:208–12.

"Will I Walk Again?"
Prognostication in Spinal Cord Compression

Paul Glare

Clinical History

A 68-year-old woman with metastatic breast cancer presents to the emergency room (ER) with a one-week history of increasing back pain, especially when getting out of bed. She also reports a 24-hour history of increasing imbalance and this morning when she woke up she discovered that she could not move her legs and she had an episode of enuresis overnight.

Examination

On examination she has a flaccid paraplegia with a sensory level above the umbilicus. Urgent MRI shows a severe spinal cord compression at T6. She is commenced on high-dose IV dexamethasone 8 mg four times a day and neurosurgery is consulted. She asks, "If have a surgery, will I be able to walk again?"

What do you tell her?

Palliative Domain of Care

Structure and Process of Care: Prognostication

When the word "prognosis" is used in the context of palliative care, the discussants are usually referring to predictions of a patient's expected survival [1]. However, forecasts can be, and are, made every day about any of the outcomes of a disease. Physicians call on their forecasting skills on a daily basis in all aspects of medicine to select treatments, prioritize diagnoses, and educate patients and families. For example, when an internist tells the patient in the office, "The chest radiograph shows you have pneumonia. I will prescribe antibiotics. You should be feeling better in a couple of days," they are utilizing their diagnostic, therapeutic, and prognostic skills [2].

In an attempt to categorize the various predictions that physicians make, the "5 D's" mnemonic was coined, which stands for:

- Death
- Disease progression or recurrence
- Disability and discomfort
- Drug toxicity
- Dollars (cost)

As with predicting death, palliative care providers need to develop expertise in formulating, communicating, and utilizing a wide range of predictions when they are caring for patients and their families.

Palliative Care Discussion

All five of the "D's" are relevant to the practice of palliative care, as illustrated by the following day-to-day interactions between palliative care physicians and patients, families, other providers, and students:

- "I can do a surgery, as long as you think he has more than three months to live."
- "The bisphosphonate will correct the calcium level but will not prevent it from recurring."
- "Unfortunately, he's unlikely to ever walk again."
- "It shouldn't make you nauseous, but if it does it usually wears off in a few days."
- "A palliative care consult will save money, by reducing unnecessary tests and treatments and shortening lengths of stay."

In fact, surveys have found that patients may be more interested in the likelihood of other outcomes than their remaining time on earth, in particular their likelihood of responding to disease-specific treatments and the side effects [3]. However, because predicted survival is so relevant to decision-making in the setting of a progressive, eventually fatal illness, much less has been written about other predictions in patients with advanced disease.

Epidural spinal cord compression (ESCC) usually arises from bone metastases in adjacent vertebrae and it typically occurs approximately two years after the onset of bone metastases [4]. At autopsy 40 percent of all patients with a history of spinal cord compression have vertebral metastases at the time of death. On MRI, almost 50 percent of patients with vertebral metastases have evidence of asymptomatic epidural disease, but the incidence of clinical ESCC is 2.5 percent of all patients. Consequently, any patient with cancer and back pain should be considered to have vertebral metastases and be at risk for ESCC until proven otherwise. The development of ESCC is really a late manifestation of cancer and survival after onset is poor, typically less than six months. It may be much shorter (less than one month) in some tumor types, e.g., gastrointestinal. Other predictors of a short survival after ESCC include a short time from cancer diagnosis to ESCC onset, and decreased ambulatory function after treatment.

Pain is the initial symptom in approximately 90 percent of patients with ESCC, and may be present for a variable amount of time, from months to just a few days. Motor weakness occurs in more than 60 percent, sensory loss in 70–80 percent, and up to 75 percent have sphincter disturbances. Neurological symptoms often develop rapidly, occurring within hours in approximately 20 percent of cases. There is variability between tumor types, with lung cancer patients having the fastest progression and the most severe functional deficits. Lung cancer patients are more likely to present with paralysis while breast cancer patients are often ambulatory. Neurological deficit is also more common when the interval between diagnosis and onset of ESCC is shorter than the average, which is approximately two years.

Functional outcomes depend on a number of factors.

- Ambulatory function before and after treatment: Mobility and bladder function at presentation is the strongest predictor of the functional outcome. Ninety percent of patients who are ambulatory at presentation will be ambulatory after treatment. In one series, only 7 percent of paralyzed patients regained full mobility (Table 6.1) and 28 percent with urinary catheters regained bladder function [5].
- The rate of development of motor symptoms: motor function is much more likely to improve when the symptoms develop slowly (over two weeks or longer).
- Pain is often not relieved in half of the patients and up to 10 percent continue to have severe pain, presumably related to the spinal cord injury.
- Extent of the epidural disease: total blockage versus partial blockage.
- The type of treatment: Treatment of ESCC includes emergent steroids, radiotherapy, and/or neurosurgery. Radiotherapy is the treatment of choice for most patients, but surgery can achieve improved outcomes in selected cases where there is spinal instability and neurological deficit. The NOMS algorithm developed at Memorial Sloan Kettering Cancer Center can aid in this decision-making [6]. Neurosurgery is also indicated in lung cancer patients with thoracic ESCC in previously irradiated fields.

Because ESCC is often a late manifestation of cancer, predicting survival has an important bearing on decision-making. Because of the time needed to recover from the operation and undergo rehab, surgery would not normally be offered to a patient with less than three months to live. Scoring systems to aid this have been developed, including the Tokashui and Tomita scores, which have an accuracy of predicting three-month survival approaching 80 percent [7]. The factors included in these scores are: primary cancer site, extent of disease, performance status, number of vertebrae with metastases, number of extra spinal bone metastases, and neurological deficit.

Hospital Course

Surgery is successful, her pain improves, and her bladder function returns to normal, but she remains unable to walk. Palliative radiotherapy is scheduled for six weeks and she is transferred to a subacute rehab facility to work on her ambulatory function.

Table 6.1 Ambulation function and outcomes in epidural spinal cord compression (based on data in [5]).

Ambulatory Function	Before Radiotherapy	After Radiotherapy	Survival
Totally paralyzed	43 percent	40 percent	One month
Move legs but can't walk	31 percent	20 percent	
Walk with assistance	19 percent	17 percent	Two to three months
Walk unaided	60 percent	76 percent	Five months

Unfortunately, this woman probably won't ever walk again. Only 13 percent of paraplegic patients will regain function after treatment for ESCC, although the outcomes may be better after surgery. Depending on her social situation, she may not be able to ever return home. Her overall prognosis is poor and she would be eligible for hospice if she decides not to opt for further cancer-directed treatment.

General Remarks

Because of the uncertainty of the future, and the complex dynamic system of the human body, predicting death and other outcomes in patients with advanced disease can seem mysterious, unknowable, and powerful. Through applying scientific methods, medicine has and can make advancements in predicting medical outcomes, despite the formidable task. A century ago, it would have been thought impossible to predict the landfall of hurricanes or the approach of a blizzard, but meteorology has begun to understand and predict the near-future outcomes of the complex dynamic system of Earth's climate. Medicine should continue to attempt the same.

Suggested Reading

1. Glare P, Sinclair C, Downing M, et al. Predicting survival in patients with advanced disease. *Eur J Cancer*. 2008;**44**:1146–56.

2. Glare PA, Sinclair CT. Palliative medicine review: prognostication. *J Palliat Med*. 2008;**11**:84–103.

3. Steinhauser KE, Christakis NA, Clipp EC, et al. Preparing for the end of life: Preferences of patients, families, physicians, and other care providers. *J Pain Symptom Manage*. 2001;**22**:727–37.

4. Hoskin PJ, Grover A, Bhana R. Metastatic spinal cord compression: Radiotherapy outcome and dose fractionation. *Radiother Oncol*. 2003;**68**:175–80.

5. Conway R, Graham J, Kidd J, et al. What happens to people after malignant cord compression? Survival, function, quality of life, emotional well-being and place of care 1 month after diagnosis. *Clin Oncol (R Coll Radiol)*. 2007;**19**:56–62.

6. Laufer I, Rubin DG, Lis E, et al. The NOMS framework: Approach to the treatment of spinal metastatic tumors. *Oncologist*. 2013;**18**:744–51.

7. Tokuhashi Y, Matsuzaki H, Oda H, et al. A revised scoring system for preoperative evaluation of metastatic spine tumor prognosis. *Spine (Phila Pa 1976)*. 2005;**30**: 2186–91.

Prolonged Grief Following the Death of a Spouse

Sue E. Morris

Clinical History

Kate is a 35-year-old woman who contacted the Cancer Center's bereavement program six months after her husband's death. Kate reported that her 38-year-old husband, John, was diagnosed with glioblastoma approximately two years before his death. At the time of his diagnosis, John was employed in the finance industry and was a devoted husband and father of two young children, now aged seven and five.

During the initial bereavement visit, Kate expressed that she was having an extremely difficult time accepting her husband's death, stating that caring for her children was the only thing that got her up each morning. She reported feeling overwhelmed, deeply saddened, and angry. Kate also said that she could not get the images of John's last months out of her mind. Her grief was palpable as she spoke of the enormity of her loss. Not only had she lost her husband, but Kate said that after her husband went home with hospice, she also lost the support of the care team whom she considered "like a second family." Kate stated that she felt sad for herself at being widowed at a young age, sad for her children growing up without their father, and sad for John because of everything that he will miss out on.

Kate was also struggling to make sense of her husband's death. She said that she felt very angry, especially about the aggressiveness of his illness, stating that "no one ever survives; you only have to google glioblastoma to find out that no one with this disease lives." She expressed anger directed toward the doctors' inability to cure her husband. "You know, you come to a place like this, one of the best in the world, and even these oncologists can't find a cure – what must it be like to work in this place and go home each night, knowing that all of your patients are going to die?"

Kate's circle of support had dwindled over the last year of her husband's life as the demands of caregiving for him increased, adding to her sense of isolation. During the course of her husband's treatment, Kate had met regularly with the team's social worker. Since John's death, she had not sought bereavement support. She had no previous psychiatric history.

Examination

Bereavement risk screening helps clinicians identify individuals potentially at risk for developing complicated or prolonged grief. By identifying risk factors, recommendations for support can be made either before or after a patient's death, ideally before. While it can be difficult to predict how an individual will cope after a death, identifying risk factors can help the clinician think systematically about potential difficulties and intervene early.

Table 7.1 lists Kate's risk factors using a simple bereavement risk-screening tool [1]. Based on her initial interview, Kate presents with four known risk factors: lack of or poor social support, concurrent stresses, high initial distress, and witnessing a difficult death. Of particular note is Kate's high level of caregiver burden. Not only did she care for her husband over the course of his illness and witness his decline, she is also a young mother with small children who require ongoing care, giving her little opportunity to address her own bereavement needs.

Kate currently meets the criteria for prolonged grief disorder (PGD) that has been proposed for ICD-11 [2]. Prolonged grief disorder is a distinct mental disorder characterized by intense, prolonged symptoms of grief that results in clinically significant impairment in functioning. The diagnosis should not be made until at least six months have elapsed since the death. The bereaved individual experiences yearning for the deceased and several disabling symptoms. In Kate's case, these symptoms include: difficulty accepting the loss, inability to trust others since her husband's death, anger related to the loss, difficulty

Table 7.1 Kate's bereavement risk screen

Risk Factor	Yes	No	Unsure
History of psychiatric disorders, including drug and alcohol use		X	
History of childhood separation anxiety			X
Lack of or poor social support	X		
Concurrent stresses	X		
Previous losses			X
High initial distress	X		
Unexpected diagnosis and unanticipated death		X	
Lack of preparation for death		X	
Dependent relationship with deceased			X
Conflict with deceased/unresolved issues		X	
Death of a child		X	
Witnessing a difficult death	X		

moving on with life, feeling that life is meaningless, and feeling shocked by the loss.

Palliative Domain of Care

Care of the Patient at the End of Life – Prolonged grief and bereavement risk screening

According to the National Consensus Project for Quality Palliative Care, this domain highlights communication and focuses on family guidance about the dying process and the post-death period [3]. Bereavement support is emphasized, including anticipatory grief in the period prior to the death with ongoing support throughout the bereavement period. As such, clinicians can play a significant role in the care of families before and after the death of a patient.

Kate received little formal psychosocial support prior to her husband's death. The majority of her support came from her interactions with her husband's care team, including meetings with a neuro-oncology social worker when possible during treatment visits. Unfortunately, as the frequency of her husband's treatment visits decreased, Kate had less contact with the social worker. Transitioning to hospice was a challenge for Kate, especially as she was very connected to the treatment team and felt somewhat abandoned by them when her husband's treatment ended.

Palliative Care Discussion

The focus of the initial bereavement visit was to assess Kate's current level of coping since her husband's death six months prior, to help her understand her experience, and to encourage her to seek professional help. Information about the wave-like nature of grief and cognitive behavioral therapy strategies that might help alleviate her suffering were outlined. The visit also provided an opportunity for Kate to tell her story, an important intervention for bereaved individuals, especially those who have little opportunity to do so within their own community. Kate's tremendous loss was acknowledged and recommendations for support were made, including joining a young widows' support group, attending individual counseling, and seeing her primary care physician.

Psychological Interventions

When working with bereaved individuals the overall aims are: (1) to help them adjust to life without the deceased, and (2) to help them maintain a connection with the deceased that is now based on memory and legacy. The first step is to assess their functioning and to gain an understanding of the circumstances surrounding the death.

Routine issues that need to be addressed include:

1. the bereaved's story
2. what they have lost with the death of their loved one
3. their social, religious, and cultural backgrounds
4. their social support network
5. past psychiatric history, including current and past use of drugs and alcohol

31

6. concurrent stressors
7. coping skills
8. unresolved or unfinished business with the deceased
9. their goals for seeking support

Applying a psycho-educational framework, strategies to help the bereaved based on self-help principles and cognitive behavior therapy [4, 5] can be grouped into six categories:

1. Education about the nature of grief and what to expect
   - Grief follows a wave-like pattern
   - Grief is unique
   - Grief is a normal response to loss that involves adaptation to change; it is not an illness with a prescribed cure

2. Opportunities to express their loss and acknowledge the death
   - Individual counseling
   - Attending a support group
   - Journal writing
   - Arranging a visit with the treatment team to have any questions answered and to say goodbye to the team and to the institution as a whole

3. Self-care activities
   - Establishing a daily routine
   - Making an appointment to see their family doctor
   - Writing a daily to-do list of what needs to be done and prioritizing
   - Daily physical activity

4. Facing new or difficult situations and tackling barriers
   - Assistance with making difficult decisions
   - Gradual exposure to situations that are difficult or avoided
   - Challenging unhelpful thoughts, especially those leading to anger or guilt
   - Making a plan for tackling "firsts"

5. Reinvesting in social connections
   - Identifying those friends or family members who have empathy and can best provide support
   - Accepting invitations to meet with friends and family even if they don't feel like it

6. Maintaining a connection with the deceased
   - Making a memory book of their life together
   - Supporting a significant cause in their memory
   - Focusing on the deceased's legacy – What did they learn from them? How would they like to be remembered? What would their loved one want for them now as they go on in their life?
   - Creating new traditions, especially around significant events such as birthdays, holidays, and anniversaries

Kate attended three individual counseling sessions at the Cancer Center, where the main focus was encouraging her to tell her story and to express her anger about the unfairness of her husband's death. One question that helped her think about her future was: "What would John want for you now?" She was able to articulate that he would want her and the children to be happy, to go out with friends, and for her to eventually have another relationship. She also realized that she would need to ask for help and was able to identify several people in her life who could provide her with support regarding her bereavement and childcare. Kate also joined a young widows' support group within her community offered by a local hospice. This group was a very important component of Kate's treatment as she began to feel less isolated as she gained support from others who were experiencing something similar. Eventually Kate was able to meet with members of her husband's treatment team to say goodbye and she accepted a referral to a community provider for longer-term therapy to deal with the traumatic memories she was experiencing.

General Remarks

The death of a significant loved one is believed to be the most powerful stressor in everyday life, placing bereaved individuals at increased risk of serious physical and mental health issues [6, 7]. While it is estimated that the majority of bereaved people cope with their losses without requiring treatment, a significant number do experience suffering from prolonged or complicated grief. Even though grief is a normal and expected response to loss, it can be an excruciatingly painful and isolating experience where adjustments can take months or even years, with great variability among individuals and across cultures [7].

From a psychological perspective, the process of grieving involves adaptation to change brought about by loss [1]. Clinicians can play a significant role in the care of families before and after the death of a patient. Before death, clinicians can help family members prepare by providing clear and accurate information about the prognosis, which facilitates decision-making, in addition to information about the dying process. Preparation for death, including an opportunity to say goodbye and being involved in end-of-life care, helps bereavement adjustment, as does an early referral to palliative care and hospice. If patients do transition to hospice care, it is recommended that a follow-up call be made by the treatment team soon after to check in with the caregiver to ease the adjustment, and to lessen potential feelings of abandonment by the team. In neurological cases, it can be helpful to have discussions with family members to acknowledge and name the multiple losses that occur as the patient's function declines. It is also important to assess their coping skills and vulnerabilities, paying attention to the risk factors for prolonged grief or other difficult bereavement outcomes as listed in Table 7.1. For those individuals who do present with risk factors, make a referral as early as possible to an appropriate community-based clinician who can help the individual address anticipatory grief. This is especially important for those family members who lack support given the isolating nature of grief.

After a death, sending a letter of condolence from either the physician or the team is an essential component of quality end-of-life care and should be incorporated as a part of routine practice. Family members benefit greatly from receiving condolence letters from clinicians. If appropriate, write something that you will miss about the patient and emphasize the good job the family member did in supporting the patient. Clinicians also benefit from the practice of writing condolence letters as it can help to process the loss and acknowledge the burden of care that is often experienced when caring for dying patients. Bereavement telephone calls also provide an opportunity to express condolences, assess coping, make recommendations for support as needed, and to say goodbye.

This case study highlights the importance of providing clear and accurate information about prognosis and disease progression to caregivers, while at the same time providing psychosocial support to help the caregiver deal with ongoing losses and anticipatory grief that frequently accompany the declining function of the patient. The case also highlights the difficulty that caregivers sometimes experience in neurological cases when treatment ends and the support from the team ceases. Early hospice referrals have been shown to improve bereavement outcomes for families [8, 9] and referrals to community providers, such as mental health clinicians and caregiver support groups, should also be recommended. Utilizing community resources early in the process creates a multilayered support system, which helps to facilitate community-based support for the caregiver once the patient stops treatment. This layered approach not only supports the caregiver during the patient's final weeks and months of life but it already is in place for the early stages of their bereavement.

Suggested Reading

1. Morris SE, Block SD. Grief and bereavement. In Grassi L, Riba M, eds. *Clinical Psycho-oncology: An International Perspective*. West Sussex: Wiley-Blackwell. 2012; 271–80.

2. Prigerson HG, Horowitz MJ, Jacobs SC, et al. Prolonged grief disorder: Psychometric validation of criteria proposed for *DSM-V* and *ICD-11*. Brayne C, ed. *PLoS Medicine*. 2009; 6(8):e1000121. doi: 10.1371/journal.pmed.1000121.

3. National Consensus Project for Quality Palliative Care. *Clinical Practice Guidelines for Quality Palliative Care, Third Edition*. Pittsburgh, PA: National Consensus Project for Quality Palliative Care. 2013.

4. Kavanagh DJ. Towards a cognitive-behavioural intervention for adult grief reactions. *British Journal of Psychiatry*. 1990;157:373–83.

5. Morris SE. *Overcoming Grief: A Self-Help Guide Using Cognitive Behavioural Techniques*. London: Constable Robinson, 2008.

6. Holmes TH, Rahe RH. The Social Readjustment Rating Scale. *Journal of Psychosomatic Research*. 1967;11:213–18.

7. Stroebe M, Schut H, Stroebe W. Health outcomes of bereavement. *Lancet*. 2007;370:1960–73. PubMed PMID: 18068517.

8. Bradley EH, Prigerson H, Carlson MD, et al. Depression among surviving caregivers: Does length of hospice enrollment matter? *Am J Psychiatry*. 2004; 161:2257–62. PubMed PMID: 15569897.

9. Christakis NA, Iwashyna TJ. The health impact of health care on families: A matched cohort study of hospice use by decedents and mortality outcomes in surviving, widowed spouses. *Soc Sci Med*. 2003;57:465–75. PubMed PMID: 12791489.

Mitigating Bereavement Risk Following a Sudden Death

Sue E. Morris

Clinical History

Mrs. C was a healthy and active 75-year-old woman who suffered a major stroke at home witnessed by her husband. Mrs. C was transported to the local hospital by ambulance, where she died three days later in the intensive care unit (ICU), never having regained consciousness.

Mr. and Mrs. C had been married for 52 years and have three children and five grandchildren. They appear to be a close and loving family. At the time of Mrs. C's stroke, her oldest daughter, Anna, was living out of state. Anna arrived at the hospital the day following her mother's stroke, but was unable to communicate with her. Anna was very shocked and upset when she saw her mother in the hospital. She was also very worried about her father and wonders whether he will be able to continue to live independently.

Anna is requesting to speak to someone from the team as she has several questions about her mother's stroke and the medical interventions that were considered. How can the team help Anna and her family prepare for Mrs. C's pending death and their bereavement?

Examination

Bereavement risk screening helps clinicians identify individuals potentially at risk of developing difficult bereavement reactions, such as prolonged grief disorder. By considering risk factors in a systematic way, recommendations for support can be made either before or after the patient's death. While it can be difficult to predict how an individual will cope after a death, there is a lot clinicians can do before the death that can help mitigate a difficult bereavement reaction.

In this case, little information is known about Anna's background. Because bereavement follow-up is often haphazard, clinicians may only have one visit with a family member to make suggestions about their bereavement care. Based on the information available, the bereavement risk-screening tool that follows can be used to help identify potential risk factors to inform interventions [1]. Table 8.1 lists Anna's known bereavement risk factors.

Table 8.1 Anna's bereavement risk screen

Risk Factor	Yes	No	Unsure
History of psychiatric disorders, including drug and alcohol use			X
History of childhood separation anxiety			X
Lack of or poor social support		X	
Concurrent stresses	X		
Previous losses			X
High initial distress	X		
Unexpected diagnosis and unanticipated death	X		
Lack of preparation for death	X		
Dependent relationship with deceased		X	
Conflict with deceased/unresolved issues		X	
Death of a child		X	
Witnessing a difficult death	X		

At this early stage, the focus from the bereavement risk screen is the prevention of a difficult bereavement outcome. It is too early to tell whether Anna or her family will have difficulty coping following Mrs. C's death, but the clinician can play an active role in helping the family prepare for Mrs. C's death and their bereavement. For Anna, potential barriers to a healthy bereavement outcome may include feelings of guilt and regret about living out of state, set within the context of her mother's unexpected death in the ICU, a factor linked to increased risk of post-traumatic stress disorder in bereaved family members [2]. Anna is also worried about her father and his adjustment, which for adult children often takes precedence over their own grief. This role reversal can bring with it increased stress for the adult child due to additional tasks and responsibilities. Early acknowledgment of these changed responsibilities can help guide discussions about accessing support.

Palliative Domain of Care

Care of the Patient at the End of Life – Unanticipated death and bereavement risk screening

According to the National Consensus Project for Quality Palliative Care, this domain highlights communication and focuses on family guidance about the dying process and the post-death period [3]. Bereavement support is emphasized, including anticipatory grief in the period prior to the death with ongoing support throughout the bereavement period. As such, clinicians can play a significant role in the care of families before and after the death of a patient.

Mrs. C's stroke and pending death were totally unexpected by her family. The suddenness of her stroke left the family little time to process the events of the days prior or to prepare for her death. They had many questions for the team about their mother's condition and whether there was any possibility that she might recover. Mrs. C's three children were particularly worried about their father, and Anna expressed regret that she lived out of state and had not seen her mother as often as she would have liked.

Palliative Care Discussion

The focus of the meetings with Anna and her family prior to her mother's death was to prepare them for the death by providing clear and factual medical information about her mother's stroke and prognosis, allowing time for them to take in the information and to ask questions. The team also needed to prepare the family for the dying process and what to expect. Because Anna arrived a day after the rest of her family, she benefited from the team reviewing what had already been discussed with her siblings and father, in an attempt to bring her up to speed. Given the unexpectedness of the situation, it was important for the team to give Anna and her family some time to process the information, and then to return to see whether they had further questions. Revisiting information helps families absorb what they are being told in a more measured way, which helps them to understand what they are facing and are likely to expect.

In these difficult conversations, families benefit most when clinicians are compassionate, express empathy, respond to emotion, provide clear information about timelines, and take the necessary time to allow family members to talk and ask questions. When meeting a family member who has just received devastating news about a loved one, a useful strategy is to ask yourself: "What does this family member need that will help ease their bereavement?"

In Anna's case, she needed:

- Accurate medical information to help her understand her mother's condition and prognosis
- To be able to ask questions and receive answers
- To express her thoughts and feelings
- To have her reactions acknowledged
- To be able to say goodbye to her mother
- To be informed about the dying process and what she might witness
- To receive practical information and support about funeral arrangements
- To receive information about grief and what to expect in the early weeks and months of her bereavement
- To find out how best to support her father and available community resources

The clinician begins the conversation with Anna by stating what he or she knows about her mother: "I understand from what your father told me, that your mother was very healthy and no one saw this coming." After this statement, the clinician pauses, allowing Anna time to respond. She is visibly upset and nods in agreement. The clinician then continues, acknowledging her emotion: "I can see that this is very upsetting and that your mother's stroke must have come as a huge shock."

The clinician also needs to help Anna prepare for her mother's death by giving accurate information: "I wish I had better news; your mother's imaging and examination indicate that she will not recover from the stroke and that we now have to focus on her end-of-life care." Again, the focus is to respond to emotion by expressing empathy and provide clear information about how much time her mother has left and what to expect during the dying process. It's also important to help Anna (and her family) prepare to say goodbye to her mother and ways that she might do this, for example, the opportunity to speak to her alone even if she can't respond. Some families also need guidance and practical information about funeral arrangements.

In the case of sudden and unexpected death, anticipate questions that might arise in the future, remembering that family members often second guess their own actions and feel guilty because they didn't "see the signs" or "act sooner." Providing factual information in simple terms helps them understand the likely cause of the death from a medical perspective. This information can also be used as "evidence" to challenge unhelpful thoughts that they might have later about feeling responsible for not being able to prevent the death.

For Anna, it was important to encourage her to seek support when she returned home, given that the reality of her mother's death could take some months to set in. She met briefly with the hospital social worker just after her mother died, who then made a bereavement call a week later. During this call, the social worker outlined the wave-like pattern of grief and what Anna might likely expect in the months ahead, especially concerning the many changes that they are now facing regarding her father's living arrangements. The social worker also encouraged Anna to contact a local hospice about attending a bereavement support group for adult children given she did not live near her siblings. Finally, the team sent separate condolence letters to Anna and Mr. C expressing their sympathy and how impressed they were in the way the family cared for Mrs. C despite how difficult the circumstances were.

Psychological Strategies

The overall aims of bereavement care are: (1) to help the bereaved adjust to life without the deceased, and (2) to help them maintain a connection with the deceased that is now based on memory and legacy.

In cases of sudden or unexpected death, bereaved individuals often struggle with unanswered questions and not having had the opportunity to say goodbye. Given the shock that often accompanies sudden death, individuals usually benefit from being able to tell their story and express their feelings over and over. Understanding what happened and making some kind of sense of it will take time and may require professional intervention.

When meeting a bereaved individual after the death, the first step is to assess their current level of functioning and to gain an understanding of the circumstances surrounding the death [1].

Routine issues that need to be addressed include:

1. the bereaved's story
2. what they have lost with the death of their loved one
3. their social, religious, and cultural backgrounds
4. their social support network
5. past psychiatric history, including current and past use of drugs and alcohol
6. concurrent stressors
7. coping skills
8. unresolved or unfinished business with the deceased
9. their goals for seeking support

In addition to attending a support group, Anna would most likely benefit from seeking counseling to address not only her own grief and any potential barriers such as guilt but also how she and her siblings could best support their father. Given she had not seen her mother recently, writing a letter telling her what she wished she could have said in person can provide an opportunity to express her thoughts and feelings. Similarly, legacy work can help recently bereaved individuals maintain a connection with the deceased. Questions to be answered include:

- What did you learn from them?
- What values did they impart to you?
- What would they want for you now and in years to come?

General Remarks

Bereavement is a normal yet complex human response to the death of a significant loved one that varies considerably among individuals and across cultures. From a psychological perspective, it involves adjusting to change brought about by loss [1]. While the majority of individuals adapt to their losses without professional intervention, grieving remains an intensely painful and isolating period for many, often lasting months or even years [4]. Given that the death of a loved one is considered the most stressful life event in everyday life [5], screening for bereavement risk as a part of routine practice facilitates early intervention.

This case highlights the role that palliative care clinicians can play, both before and after the death of a patient, in preventing a difficult bereavement following an unexpected death. Providing clear and accurate information in a compassionate way about the medical condition of the patient, typical outcomes, and also information about the dying process can help families prepare emotionally and to make plans. Responding to emotion and providing family members the opportunity to ask questions can help calm them at a time of a great distress. Post-loss, family members sometimes fall prey to the bias of hindsight, believing that they could have or should have done something to change the course of events. These beliefs can lead to feelings of anger and guilt that potentially result in difficulties. Cognitive behavior therapy strategies can help individuals challenge these unhelpful thoughts [6].

Providing scientific facts about the medical condition and its usual outcomes helps families process information that can be especially difficult in cases like Mrs. C's, where there is little time to prepare. Inviting families to return to the hospital at a later date to review information or to ask additional questions helps them to further process the loss.

Encouraging individuals to seek bereavement support within the early months following a sudden death is good practice given that sudden death is a known risk factor for prolonged or complicated grief [7]. Clinicians who have formed a therapeutic alliance at the time of the death are in a unique position to make such a recommendation.

Suggested Reading

1. Morris SE, Block SD. Grief and bereavement. In Grassi L, Riba M, eds. *Clinical Psycho-oncology: An International Perspective*. West Sussex: Wiley-Blackwell. 2012; 271–80.

2. Wright AA, Keating NL, Balboni TA, et al. Place of death: Correlations with quality of life of patients with cancer and predictors of bereaved caregivers' mental health. *J Clin Oncol*. 2010;**28**:4457–64. doi: 10.1200/JCO.2009.26.3863. PubMed PMID: 20837950; PubMed Central PMCID: PMC2988637.

3. National Consensus Project for Quality Palliative Care. *Clinical Practice Guidelines for Quality Palliative Care, Third Edition*. Pittsburgh: National Consensus Project for Quality Palliative Care. 2013.

4. Stroebe M, Schut H, Stroebe W. Health outcomes of bereavement. *Lancet*. 2007;**370**:1960–73. PubMed PMID: 18068517.

5. Holmes TH, Rahe RH. The Social Readjustment Rating Scale. Journal of Psychosomatic Research 1967;**11**:213–18.

6. Morris SE. *Overcoming Grief: A Self-Help Guide Using Cognitive Behavioural Techniques*. London: Constable Robinson. 2008.

7. Lobb EA, Kristjanson LJ, Aoum, SM, et al. Predictors of complicated grief: A systematic review of empirical studies. *Death Studies*. 2010;**34**:673–98.

"I'm Praying for a Miracle"

Priscilla H. Howick and Maisha T. Robinson

Clinical History

A 67-year-old man with a history of diabetes mellitus and hypertension was transferred to our hospital for further management of a left middle cerebral artery territory stroke after receiving intravenous tissue plasminogen activator (IV-tPA).

Earlier in the day, he had told his wife that he wasn't feeling well. He felt a general sense of weakness, which prompted him to lie down for a nap. Upon waking, he felt better and they went to their church for a conference. While at the event, he was initially able to engage in the planned activities, but during the course of the evening, his wife looked over at him and she noticed that he had a right facial droop and that the entire right side of his body was "dead weight." He was unable to speak. Emergency medical services were called and he was taken to the local hospital, where he received IV-tPA. His National Institute of Stroke Scale score was 32. He was transferred to our hospital intubated for possible neurosurgical endovascular intervention. Upon arrival, a CT angiogram revealed matched perfusion defects, suggesting that there was no salvageable brain tissue. He remained globally aphasic and hemiplegic in the neurologic intensive care unit for 10 days. A repeat head CT showed a large left MCA territory stroke with malignant edema and 4 mm midline shift. The palliative medicine team was consulted to clarify goals of care with his wife, a woman of great faith who pastored a church in their hometown.

Palliative Domain of Care

Spiritual Aspects of Care

Palliative care consultations focus on not only the physical or psychological symptoms that patients or families may encounter when dealing with a serious medical illness but also the spiritual beliefs that may influence goals of care and management plans. Obtaining a spiritual history involves more than identifying whether a patient has a faith tradition or an affiliation with a specific religious community.

The discussion is broadened to be inclusive of what gives the patient purpose and meaning and what aspects of their belief system may assist in the coping process or guide decisions about care.

Palliative Care Discussion

Spirituality is important to many patients and surrogate decision makers who are facing serious medical conditions. Despite this, the topic is infrequently broached by the medical team, even in intensive care settings where a patient's belief system may impact medical decision-making about life-sustaining interventions or quality of life issues.

In this case, the patient and her husband's faith tradition was Inter-denominational. His wife was a pastor of a small church and they had recently completed a three-week period of fasting and praying with their congregation. During the consultation, she mentioned that she knew the Lord was preparing them for something but she couldn't have known that it would be this situation. Her family and her church were praying for her husband's recovery and she was praying for a miracle.

Hospital Course

The palliative care team met with the patient's wife to help her understand the gravity of the situation and to discuss treatment goals. The team started by asking her understanding of her husband's condition, and she responded that his condition is "not good," and she feared he may "not be able to recover" from the stroke. She added, "But … I know that God can heal him."

PALLIATIVE MEDICINE PHYSICIAN (PMP) – Mrs. H, what are you hoping for your husband?

MRS. H – I'm hoping he will wake up and get off that breathing machine.

CHAPLAIN – Yes, that is always the hope we feel in our hearts. We also would like very much for that to happen.

Unfortunately, Mrs. H, given your husband's condition, we don't think that will happen. Your husband's body ... his brain ... has been severely compromised. He may not be able to wake up and come off the breathing machine.

Mrs. H – God can do anything.

PMP – We believe that too, and we recognize that we may be interfering with divine will.

Chaplain – Did your husband ever talk about his wishes if something like this were to happen?

Mrs. H – No, but I know he would want to be kept alive.

PMP – Did he ever talk about being kept alive if he could not walk, or talk, or interact with his loved ones?

Mrs. H – No, he didn't.

Chaplain – Mrs. H, while the decision is a difficult one, have you considered that it may be best for your husband if we move out of the way and allow him to die a natural, peaceful death? In his current state, he cannot make that decision for himself. It's up to you to allow him to release from his body and go be with the Lord.

Mrs. H – If God wants him (husband), I believe he can come down from Heaven and unplug the machine himself.

The team recognized how deeply the patient's wife was suffering. Plans were made to return the following day to continue the conversation.

Subsequent visits by the chaplain revealed that Mrs. H's stance was informed by her belief that if she agreed to withdraw life-prolonging care, she would be held accountable by God for the death of her husband; she felt she would be killing him. Attempts to help her reframe this belief were met with her fear and anxiety about being responsible for the decision to compassionately wean him from the ventilator.

General Remarks

Sometimes, as this case demonstrates, two cultures come into conflict and make it difficult for patients and families to get on the same page with the medical team in terms of treatment goals. One culture is driven by evidence-based clinical judgment that allows a reasonable determination of outcomes. The other culture is influenced by religious belief and embraces the possibility that a power higher than medical science can intervene and bring a desired result. The stance of "waiting for the miracle" gives rise to possibility and often rubs up against medical

judgment, which is based on probability. How, then, can these two seemingly opposite views be reconciled? Sometimes they cannot; however, any hope of moving toward a working relationship requires communication that seeks to understand the frame of reference of the individuals involved. Religion and faith develop along a spectrum and the psychology of faith may add insight into this case.

Developmental psychologist James Fowler suggests there are six stages of faith development. Based on work by Jean Piaget, Erik Erikson, and Lawrence Kolberg, Fowler observed that just as a child evolves from concrete literal thinking to more complex cognitive constructs, so does their understanding of faith.

Fowler states:
Questions of faith are aimed at helping us get in touch with the dynamic, patterned process by which we find life meaningful. They aim to help us reflect on the centers of value and power that sustain our lives; the persons, causes and institutions we really love and trust, the images of good and evil, of possibility and probability to which we are committed – these form the pattern of our faith [1].

Faith is not always religious in its content or context, though it is often easier to identify when religious content is present, as in this case. It can be observed universally that faith follows these stages. For purposes of this chapter, we are not able to list all six stages; however, it is pertinent to note that the wife in this case was operating from Fowler's "Synthetic-Conventional" faith stage (arising in adolescence; aged 12 to adulthood), characterized by conformity to authority and the religious development of a personal identity. Any conflicts with one's beliefs are ignored at this stage due to the threat that arises from inconsistency in beliefs. For Mrs. H, the threat of losing her husband was too great to assimilate into her reality. She chose to cling to her belief that "God can do anything" in order to alleviate her anxiety about her husband dying. At some point, as Mrs. H faces the reality of her husband's death, she will have to find a way to reconcile the gap between her belief in a miracle and the absence of one. In addition, Mrs. H has to reconcile her belief that deciding to discontinue the ventilator is equal to actively killing her husband.

Often what transitions one into the next stage of faith development is a crisis whereby one is thrown into spiritual distress, a disruption in one's belief system. In the fourth stage of faith development, one begins to critically examine beliefs and often can become disillusioned, forcing one to reconstruct beliefs to fit life experience. One starts to see outside the box of one's worldview and realizes there are other boxes. As the individual works through the distress, they begin to demonstrate stage 5 characteristics, accepting that life has mystery and is filled with paradox. In the fifth stage, one's faith is not challenged when the miracle does not come in the way they hoped. Instead one can reframe the miracle and find new meaning, such as, the idea that their loved one did not suffer. This faith stance tends to be more resilient in the face of challenging life experience.

In this case, the palliative team sought to partner with Mrs. H and validate her belief system while remaining realistic and honest about her husband's prognosis. Further exploration by the chaplain revealed that Mrs. H had several psychosocial-spiritual issues that greatly influenced her decision-making. First and foremost, she did not want the responsibility for making the decision to remove her husband from the ventilator. In her system of belief, this decision belongs to God alone and she did not want to live the rest of her life with the moral guilt of thinking she had killed her husband. Mrs. H also worried that her community of faith might view her decision negatively and that this could lead to her being ostracized from her support system. In addition, the death of her husband meant she would now have to shoulder many responsibilities once managed by her husband. Making the decision to discontinue life-sustaining care was too great for her to assimilate in such a short time. She needed more time to adjust to the mounting changes that were overwhelming her as she anticipated the loss of her beloved husband.

This case demonstrates that the issues involved are often complex and multifaceted and require intention to bring to awareness. Patients and their caregivers struggle with spiritual issues that underlie and drive many of the problems that arise in the emotional, social, and even physical domains of care. Palliative means to anticipate, assess, and alleviate suffering in all the domains of care, including the spiritual.

Mrs. H found refuge in her faith during a time when she felt alone and overwhelmed. Hoping for a miracle was her way of coping and it provided relief, comfort, and peace in the midst of her emotional upheaval. Exercising her faith and trust in God helped to alleviate her suffering when her foundations were being shaken. The chaplain was able to validate her faith and invite her into deeper exploration even as she wrestled with her spiritual distress. This in turn provided insight for the palliative team, who was then able to address her fears and needs. Mrs. H was not able to make the decision to compassionately wean her husband from the ventilator. That decision required a level of courage that she was not able to provide for herself or her husband. She was, however, able to accept the reality of her husband's imminent death, and she was a little less fragmented when he died several days later.

Acknowledging a patient or family member's belief system creates a partnership that can open up communication and shed light on what influences decision-making. Discounting belief systems creates a power struggle that diminishes communication and closes opportunity for collaboration. When managing the patient or family waiting for the miracle, it is important to listen and explore religious values and what is driving their decision-making. Inquiring about one's faith out of compassion and a desire to understand is much different than questioning one's faith from a place of judgment and criticism. It is important to recognize that asking about one's faith does not take a great deal of time and listening will give insight into decision-making. When possible, it is good to invite to the table a professional board-certified chaplain who is trained in exploring beliefs and who can often help reframe a situation in the context of religious faith that is true to both cultures.

Suggested Reading

1. Ernecoff NC, Curlin FA, Buddadhumaruk P, White DB. Health care professionals' responses to religious or spiritual statements by surrogate decision makers during goals-of-care discussions. *JAMA Intern Med.* 2015 Oct;**175**(10):1662–9.

2. Fowler, James W. (1976). *Stages of Faith: The Psychology of Human Development and the Question of Meaning.* San Francisco, CA: Harper and Row Publishers.

3. Pulaski C, Ferrell B, Virani R, Otis-Green S, Baird P, Bull J, Chochinov H, Handzo G, Nelson-Becker H, Prince-Paul M, Pugliese K, Sulmasy D. Improving the quality of spiritual care as a dimension of palliative care: the report of the Consensus Conference. *J Palliat Med.* 2009:**12**(10):885.

"Should His Devices Be Deactivated?"

Shayna Rich and Maisha T. Robinson

Clinical History

A 69-year-old man with a history of ischemic heart disease with subsequent congestive heart failure, which required placement of a pacemaker/cardiac defibrillator (ICD) and left ventricular assist device (LVAD) as a bridge to transplant, developed slurred speech and confusion approximately four months after the LVAD was placed. A non-contrast head CT revealed subacute left thalamic and medial occipital lobe infarctions with mild hemorrhagic conversion (Figure 10.1). His international normalized ratio (INR) on hospital admission was 2.3, lactate dehydrogenase was 240. The stroke mechanism was likely embolic secondary to the LVAD. He was maintained on warfarin

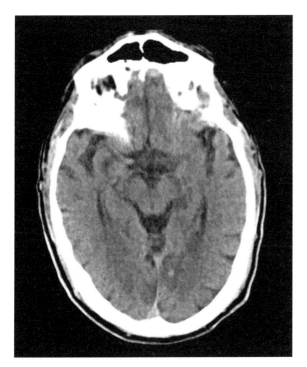

Figure 10.1 Non-contrast CT head showing left occipital infarct

and aspirin during his hospital stay. At the time of discharge to an inpatient rehabilitation facility four days after his stroke, his neurological exam was remarkable for a right lower quadrant visual deficit, mild ataxia of the right upper extremity, and expressive aphasia. As a result of his stroke, he was taken off of the transplant list.

Following rehabilitation, he was seen as an outpatient by neurology. At that time, his wife described frequent episodes of confusion and continued difficulty getting his words out. Since his discharge from the rehabilitation facility, he had required constant redirection at home as he engaged in his activities of daily living (ADLs). On examination, he had a residual aphasia and the mental status examination was notable for disorientation and perseveration. His affect was flat.

Over the following two months, he experienced further cognitive decline. His memory worsened, he was no longer able to follow complex commands, and he required more assistance with his ADLs. A repeat CT head showed no acute changes. He underwent neuropsychological testing and he was diagnosed with cognitive impairment related to his vascular disease.

Three weeks later, he presented to the emergency department with worsening aphasia and increased agitation. He had been very restless throughout the previous 24 hours, described as pulling at objects and picking at his clothing. No acute changes were noted on imaging.

Examination

He was afebrile, hypotensive (91/72), and tachycardic (heart rate 111). He was awake and alert, and unreliably able to answer questions with one-word responses. He appeared agitated, picking at his hospital gown and grabbing nearby objects.

Palliative Domain of Care

Care of the Patient at the End of Life – Decision-making about life-sustaining treatment, including discontinuation of a defibrillator or ventricular assist device

Prior to the placement of his LVAD, the patient had completed a palliative care consultation that included a discussion of his treatment preferences if he developed a serious complication. He had specified to his wife that in the event of a catastrophic event related to his LVAD, including a stroke, he did not want to "live and be a burden to his family." He specified that in the event of a devastating stroke, he would want the LVAD deactivated and he would want to be allowed to have a natural death. He completed an advance directive form that included the designation of a health care surrogate and a living will.

Palliative Care Discussion

The patient's wife felt overwhelmed with his condition. Although he had suffered prior strokes, he had recovered sufficiently to be able to perform his ADLs with only minor assistance. His wife understood that he did not want to remain supported by the LVAD if he developed a catastrophic or life-threatening complication, but she felt more uncertain about what he would want in the setting of a series of smaller events. She had not considered the possibility that he might undergo a gradual decline related to his strokes, and she was uncertain about under what circumstances he would want his LVAD or ICD discontinued. She was hopeful that his cognitive status would improve and that he would continue to enjoy a relatively independent quality of life.

Hospital Course

The patient's aphasia returned to baseline, but he exhibited continued agitation. He was able to return home with a plan for outpatient support, including physical therapy, occupational therapy, and speech therapy.

Approximately three weeks later, he awakened in the middle of the night with a left facial droop, left hemiplegia, and confusion that was worse than his baseline. His wife was awakened by his scratching and by gurgling noises. She noted that his right hand and right foot were shaking. He was alert but unable to follow commands. Emergency medical services

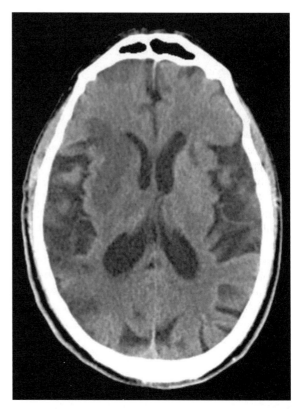

Figure 10.2 Non-contrast head CT showing interval infarctions in the right corpus striatum and the internal capsule

were called and he was transported to the emergency department for seizure management.

A non-contrast head CT revealed interval infarctions in the right basal ganglia (Figure 10.2). Over the following day, his left-sided weakness improved, but he remained confused. He developed increasing somnolence over the next few days and he was limited in his ability to participate in speech, occupational, and physical therapy. Given his cognitive and functional decline over the previous several months, his family decided to discontinue his ICD but maintain his LVAD to allow him to recover as much as possible. He became more alert after a few days and he was able to be discharged to a rehabilitation facility.

General Remarks

Patients with LVADs are at an increased risk of pump thromboses and therefore, they must be maintained on anticoagulation. As a result, they may develop neurological complications, including hemorrhagic or embolic strokes. It is important to ensure that patients are aware of this risk prior to LVAD placement, as part of the informed consent process for treatment.

In the United States, the Centers for Medicare and Medicaid Services (CMS) require the involvement of a palliative care team in the process of LVAD evaluation, although the level of this involvement varies by institution. If patients are evaluated for LVAD preparedness by a palliative care team, emphasis should be placed on: (1) ensuring that patients understand the significant risk of complications after LVAD placement, especially if the LVAD is planned as destination therapy; (2) discussing preferences for care, including any circumstances under which the LVAD should be discontinued; and (3) engaging in advance care planning, including documentation of health care surrogates and treatment preferences in case the patient becomes incapable of decision-making.

Care for patients with LVADs who develop a stroke is complicated by the need to maintain anticoagulation while limiting the risk of hemorrhagic conversion or an additional hemorrhage. Patients and families should be made aware of this delicate balance and understand that patients with a prior neurological complication are at higher risk of a second event. Neurological recovery may follow a similar time course as other stroke patients, and in many cases, rehabilitation should be offered to maximize functional recovery.

Withdrawal of life-sustaining care, including discontinuation of ICDs and LVADs, has been consistently declared legal and ethical. Patients whose treatment goals are consistent with comfort may choose to discontinue these interventions. If patients are unable to make decisions based on their neurological status, their families should consider their wishes and treatment goals when making decisions. They should understand that discontinuation of an ICD will not result in imminent death, but will only ensure that no shock will be given if the patient's heart develops an arrhythmia. The pacemaker function of any combined ICD will continue.

LVAD patients will usually live a short time, minutes to hours, following discontinuation of their LVAD. Often, this decision will be made by family members after a patient has developed a catastrophic complication. Family members may struggle with the decision about whether to discontinue the patient's LVAD support, even if the patient's preferences were clearly stated. Emotional support should be provided to clarify that the patient will be dying from the natural process of heart failure. An effort should be made to ensure that all family members who wish to be present are available prior to discontinuing the LVAD. The LVAD alarm should be turned off prior to deactivating it, and patients should be given medications as needed to maintain comfort. It may be helpful to refer patients to hospice to provide bereavement support for these families as well.

Suggested Reading

1. Dunlay SM, Strand JJ, Wordingham SE, et al. Dying with a left ventricular assist device as destination therapy. *Circ Heart Fail*. 2016 Oct;**9**(10).

2. Gafford EF, Luckhardt AJ, Swetz KM. Deactivation of a left ventricular assist device at the end of life #269. *J Palliat Med*. 2013 Aug;**16**(8):980–2.

3. Mueller PS, Swetz KM, Freeman MR, et al. Ethical analysis of withdrawing ventricular assist device support. *Mayo Clin Proc*. 2010 Sep;**85**(9): 791–7.

"Is It Time for Hospice?"

Shayna Rich and Maisha T. Robinson

Clinical History

A 40-year-old woman was diagnosed with isocitrate dehydrogenase-1 (IDH-1) wild-type anaplastic astrocytoma in the right frontal lobe after a generalized tonic-clonic seizure, and she underwent resection followed by external beam radiation therapy and concurrent temozolomide. She developed transaminitis, which led to premature discontinuation of temozolomide and adjuvant temozolomide was not provided. She remained on observation.

Approximately six months after her initial treatment course, she had another seizure and radiographic evidence of tumor progression (Figure 11.1).

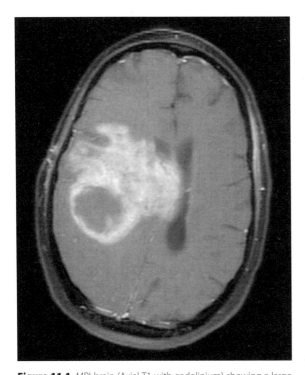

Figure 11.1 MRI brain (Axial T1 with gadolinium) showing a large right frontal heterogeneously enhancing mass with associated hemorrhage, vasogenic edema, near effacement of the right lateral ventricle, and 9 mm right to left midline shift

She was treated with single-agent bevacizumab. Over the next few months, her symptoms and imaging continued to worsen. She underwent a subtotal resection of her tumor and pathology revealed an epidermal growth factor receptor (EGFR)-positive glioblastoma. Her disease continued to progress despite treatment courses with temozolomide, followed by lomustine and bevacizumab, and a second course of external beam radiation therapy. These treatments continued for several months.

She presented to the emergency department with a few days of confusion and disorientation. On the day of presentation, she was staring into space. Her family noticed a left gaze deviation and slow responses to questions. A head CT showed the right frontal mass with worsening vasogenic edema and right-to-left subfalcine herniation (Figure 11.2).

Examination

She was awake and alert, oriented to self and year, but not to date or place. She had mild inattention during the history and examination. There was mild facial asymmetry with flattening of the left nasolabial fold. She had increased tone in all extremities, more prominent on the left with spasticity in the left upper extremity. She had 3+ reflexes on the left.

Palliative Domain of Care

Care of the Patient at the End of Life – Decision-making about hospice enrollment

The patient was unable to provide much information, as she was very somnolent and disoriented. Her husband provided most information and he hoped to avoid detailed discussions in front of the patient. She and her husband had previously avoided explicit discussion of diagnosis and prognosis. They had been told that she was dying during a previous episode six months earlier, but she had bounced back with

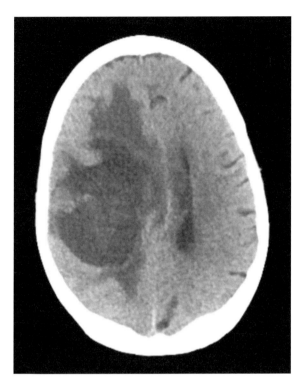

Figure 11.2 Non-contrast head CT showing a large right frontal mass with increased vasogenic edema and midline shift

steroids, and the family hoped that this episode would have a similar outcome. Their goals of care included hoping for more time with their young children with the best quality of life possible.

Her husband struggled with recognizing her functional decline since her previous hospitalization, although her mother strongly stated that she was overall worse. They both acknowledged daily fluctuations, but her husband focused on her intermittent periods of alertness. Her husband hoped that her clinical status would improve if her nutrition increased, and that she would be able to restart chemotherapy soon.

Throughout the visit, the patient did not actively participate in the discussion, but she was obviously listening. When asked direct questions at the end of the visit, she was able to simply state her preferences. She indicated that she had understood the conversation. She was hoping to return home soon, with support from home health or hospice care depending on her clinical needs. Additionally, she acknowledged her depression and stated that she would like to try an antidepressant.

Palliative Care Discussion

The patient had previously stated a desire to avoid discussion of prognosis, which limited her ability to plan for an appropriate referral to hospice. Despite our attempts to acknowledge her recent decline in cognitive and functional status, her husband was only willing to note a plateau. The patient's mother was clearly able to state that she had declined in her activity and in her ability to participate in her daily care. Her mother's observations were consistent with the worsening brain imaging, which demonstrated progression of her disease.

Given her prior episode of being told she was dying, it was reasonable that the family struggled to trust the medical team. They wanted to optimize her care and determine if she could recover with appropriate support and treatment. However, it was critical to ensure that the patient was given sufficient information for decision-making and that she was included in the discussion as much as possible. Although she appeared to be disengaged and drowsy, her level of understanding of her clinical situation was evident as she was able to express her preferences for care at the end of the discussion.

Treatment Course

The patient received a nasogastric tube for temporary supplementation of nutritional intake and was discharged home. After being home with home health, including tube feedings, for approximately one week, she chose to enter hospice. She died at home two weeks after discharge.

General Remarks

Families of patients with a limited life expectancy will often try to protect their loved ones by requesting that providers not have an open discussion of prognosis in front of the patient. Patients should always be asked directly about whether they want to have a full discussion of diagnosis and prognosis. If patients wish to limit the health information provided, that wish should be respected. Otherwise, discussions should attempt to include patients in an open way.

Patients will often understand that they have a limited prognosis and they may be protecting their family and friends in turn. It is often helpful to initiate conversation by asking about their knowledge of their disease. Patients should be encouraged to state this understanding, to break the ice. This allows everyone to participate in an open discussion that acknowledges the medical realities and that reduces anxieties for the patient and the family.

Patients and families should be encouraged to structure the discussion in the context of their experience of the disease process. Patients who are nearing their end-of-life period will usually have an increasing symptom burden and worsening clinical status. By focusing on their experience of disease, rather than scan or test results, their personal experience can be acknowledged. Patients and families will generally have an intuitive understanding of the course of the disease, and it is important for this understanding to be supported. The attendant feelings can also be normalized.

Patients should be encouraged to define their goals of care in the context of their current disease status. Although many patients are hoping to be cured, most can understand the need to develop a set of goals beyond cure, especially in the case that cure is unlikely. Patients may choose to continue to focus on extending their life as long as possible, regardless of quality, or they may choose to focus on comfort or spending time with loved ones. In either case, it is important to discuss what would be considered realistic expectations. This permits appropriate planning for additional care, and it reduces the risk of regretting decisions at the end of life. Hope should not be extinguished, but discussion should encourage setting of realistic hopes within the constraints of a patient's mortality.

Hospice care should be discussed if a patient indicates a goal of comfort care or other compatible goal (e.g., spending time at home with family and friends). A clear discussion of hospice care should include a general explanation of the care that they typically provide. Patients and families often have misunderstandings about hospice care. One common misunderstanding is that hospice care is only provided in an institution rather than at home. It is also important to explain that hospice care is not designed to shorten life expectancy, but rather allows the natural course of death to proceed. Many patients have significant fear about the process of hospice care, and a short discussion with a trusted provider can have dramatic effects on reassuring them that hospice is not designed to neglect the patient or to ensure their rapid death. It may also be helpful to ask about the patient and family's prior experiences with hospice care, if any.

Suggested Reading

1. Gunten CF. Discussing hospice care #38. *J Clin Oncol.* 2002;**20**:1419–24.
2. Hudson PL, Aranda S, Kristjanson LJ. Meeting the supportive needs of family caregivers in palliative care: Challenges for health professionals. *J Palliat Med.* 2004 Jul;7(1):19–25.
3. Whitney SN, McCullough LB, Fruge E, et al. Beyond breaking bad news: The roles of hope and hopefulness. *Cancer.* 2008 Jul 15;**113**(2):442–5.

Acute neurologic deterioration in patients with ischemic stroke, intracranial hemorrhage, or traumatic brain injuries presents a unique challenge as many of these patients were previously healthy. Approximately 70 percent of patients who are admitted to the Neurologic Intensive Care Unit previously had no medical conditions [1]. As a result, advance care planning may not have occurred prior to the event. Therefore, caregivers and health care surrogates have a critical role in clarifying the goals of care based on information from the neurological or medical teams and from their knowledge of the patient. They are tasked with making complex decisions regarding the desired level of care, often without the benefit of prior conversations addressing the patient's preferences and based on, at times, limited prognostic information [2]. Palliative care needs in the neurological intensive care unit primarily focus on identifying goals of care, providing support to caregivers and families, and assisting with coping strategies [3, 4].

In retrospective studies of neurologic patients who were evaluated by palliative care teams, common diagnoses include ischemic strokes and intracranial hemorrhage [5, 6]. The reason for palliative care consultation was more commonly related to issues regarding life-prolonging care versus symptom management. These patients often had marked functional, communication, or cognitive impairments and they commonly died in the hospital or in hospice care [5–7]. Other post-stroke palliative needs include physical and emotional symptoms, including pain, fatigue, and mood disorders [8, 9]. Palliative care should be available for all stroke patients and it may be provided by the primary medicine or neurology team, or by a specialized palliative medicine service [2, 4].

Palliative Concepts at the Time of Diagnosis: Disease-Specific Considerations

- Stroke
  - Advance directives
  - Tracheostomy/PEG
  - Accommodations for mobility impairment or cognitive dysfunction
  - Symptom management
  - Caregiver support
  - General considerations:
    · Discussion regarding the disease
    · Symptom management
    · Mood and coping
    · Progression of disease/disease trajectory
    · Advance care planning

Suggested Reading

1. Frontera JA, Curtis JR, Nelson JE, et al. Integrating palliative care into the care of neurocritically ill patients: A report from the Improving Palliative Care in the ICU Project Advisory Board and the Center to Advance Palliative Care. *Critical Care Medicine*. 2015;**43**(9): 1964–77.

2. Creutzfeldt CJ, Holloway RG, Curtis JR. Palliative care: A core competency for stroke neurologists. *Stroke*. 2015;**46**(9):2714–19.

3. Creutzfeldt CJ, Engelberg RA, Healey L, et al. Palliative care needs in the neuro-ICU. *Critical Care Medicine*. 2015;**43**(8):1677–84.

4. Tran LN, Back AL, Creutzfeldt CJ. Palliative care consultations in the neuro-ICU: A qualitative study. *Neurocritical Care*. 2016;**25**(2):266–72.

5. Holloway RG, Ladwig S, Robb J, Kelly A, Nielsen E, Quill TE. Palliative care consultations in hospitalized stroke patients. *Journal of Palliative Medicine*. 2010;**13**(4):407–12.

6. Liu Y, Kline D, Aerts S, et al. Inpatient palliative care for neurological disorders: Lessons from a large retrospective series. *Journal of Palliative Medicine.* 2017;**20**(1):59–64.

7. Chahine LM, Malik B, Davis M. Palliative care needs of patients with neurologic or neurosurgical conditions. *European Journal of Neurology.* 2008;**15**(12):1265–72.

8. Burton CR, Payne S, Addington-Hall J, Jones A. The palliative care needs of acute stroke patients: A prospective study of hospital admissions. *Age and Ageing.* 2010;**39**(5):554–9.

9. Creutzfeldt CJ, Holloway RG, Walker M. Symptomatic and palliative care for stroke survivors. *Journal of General Internal Medicine.* 2012;**27**(7):853–60.

Chapter

12

Temporary Noninvasive Ventilation in a Do-Not-Intubate Patient

Jennifer E. Fugate

Clinical History

A 94-year-old woman with a history of hypertension and hyperlipidemia was found in bed by her husband poorly responsive with left hemiparesis. She had been well before going to bed the prior evening. Paramedics were called and arrived to find her minimally responsive with left hemiparesis, irregular tachycardia, and intermittent oxygen desaturations. Paramedics asked family members if code status was known, and they were told that she was Do-Not-Resuscitate (DNR) and Do-Not-Intubate (DNI). With positioning of her airway, they were able to maintain adequate oxygen saturations and she was taken to the emergency department for evaluation. On arrival she was stuporous and in atrial fibrillation with a rapid ventricular response. Laboratory studies revealed acute kidney injury and a respiratory acidosis. A head CT revealed a large right middle cerebral artery (MCA) territory infarction (Figure 12.1). She was started on noninvasive pressure ventilation (NPPV) in the emergency department and admitted to the neuroscience intensive care unit (ICU).

Examination

She was afebrile, in atrial fibrillation with rapid ventricular response (116 beats per minute), and tachypneic (26 breaths per minute). Blood pressure was normal. She was supported with NPPV with mask in place. She was drowsy with eye opening to tactile stimulation. She had marked dysarthria, left hemineglect, and flaccid left hemiplegia.

Palliative Domains of Care

Physical Aspects of Care

The patient was tachypneic and appeared in mild respiratory distress. Dyspnea is a distressing symptom and initiation of NPPV – a supportive therapy – resulted in improvement in her respiratory distress.

Ethical and Legal Aspects of Care

The patient was unable to speak for herself when she was found by her husband. On their arrival, paramedics sought information to determine the patient's preference for level of care. The patient's family members were aware of an advance directive that the patient had filled out, and they were aware that she

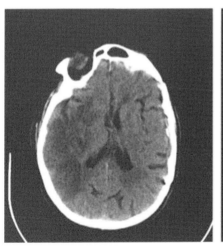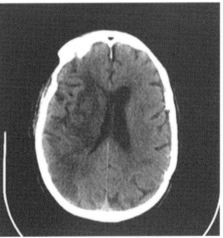

Figure 12.1 Axial non-contrast head CT showing a large right middle cerebral artery (MCA) territory infarction

had chosen her code status to be DNI/DNR. The paramedics and emergency department physicians were then able to avoid intubation, which otherwise would have been medically indicated.

There were no details about the patient's preferences regarding NPPV in her advance directive. The patient's surrogate decision makers, in collaboration with the clinicians in the emergency department, decided that the patient would receive the NPPV to alleviate dyspnea, at least for the short term.

Palliative Care Discussion

The availability of the patient's advance directive and the fact that her family was aware of the existence and contents of this document allowed the medical team members to respect the patient's goals, preferences, and choices in regards to endotracheal intubation. The use of NPPV had not been discussed in the advance directive, and its use as a palliative treatment is not always a clear decision. Dyspnea is an extremely distressing symptom and in the context of a potentially reversible etiology of respiratory failure in a patient who is DNI, it may be reasonable to pursue. In this case, respiratory failure was thought to be in part related to rapid atrial fibrillation, diastolic dysfunction, and flash pulmonary edema. Therefore, it was thought that with medical treatment and control of atrial fibrillation, this may be a reversible cause of respiratory failure. Several family members were expected to travel to the hospital to visit with the patient and the use of NPPV allowed stabilization and provided additional time for the family members to arrive.

Hospital Course

The patient was medically stabilized and remained on NPPV overnight in the ICU. Atrial fibrillation converted to normal sinus rhythm with administration of beta blockers. Her respiratory function improved considerably and by the following morning, NPPV was successfully discontinued. She was breathing regularly without distress or oxygen desaturations. She remained with a severe right middle cerebral artery stroke syndrome. A review of her advance directive indicated that she would not want any life-prolonging measures in the event of a neurologically devastating event. Her family members and the multidisciplinary medical team discussed the possibility of placing a percutaneous gastrostomy tube and all unanimously agreed that this would not be in keeping with the patient's premorbid wishes. Goals of care were transitioned to focus on her comfort and she died after several days of supportive care.

General Remarks

This patient had clear, documented preferences in her advance directive that guided her health care surrogates to make decisions in the face of a severely disabling stroke. The decisions about whether to intubate the patient or proceed with percutaneous gastrostomy tube can be challenging for family members if goals and preferences have not been clearly defined. These premorbid choices and decisions were clear and gave family members peace of mind while making them.

While those two decisions were relatively straightforward, the decision about whether to institute NPPV in a patient who is DNI is much less clear. For patients with reversible etiologies of respiratory failure, it is becoming more commonly used. In addition to temporizing the medical condition while respecting the patient's desire to not be intubated, it may also allow time for family to travel and say their goodbyes, as it did in this case. In addition, it can relieve patients from the extremely distressing symptom of dyspnea. However, it is worth noting that if the respiratory failure is not reversible, the use of NPPV may become burdensome in such a situation. Without a clearly defined endpoint (e.g., a specific time-limited trial), the NPPV mask may have the potential to prolong the dying process and perhaps also the patient's suffering by introducing new problems. A patient who requires continuous NPPV may not be able to eat well, may have difficulty communicating, and may find the mask uncomfortable. Many do not think that NPPV should be offered as a prolonged treatment in an irreversible situation for these reasons. Yet it may be appropriate with well-defined, patient-centered goals for the short term, particularly for potentially reversible causes of respiratory failure.

Suggested Reading

Alonso A, Ebert AD, Dorr D, et al. End-of-life decisions in acute stroke patients: An observational cohort study. *BMC Palliat Care.* 2016;**15**:38.

Borasio GD. The role of palliative care in patients with neurological diseases. *Nat Rev Neurol.* 2013;**9**:292–5.

Creutzfeldt CJ, Holloway RG, Curtis JR. Palliative care: A core competency for stroke neurologists. *Stroke*. 2015;**46**: 2714–19.

Frontera JA, Curtis JR, Nelson JE, et al. Integrating palliative care into the care of neurocritically ill patients: A report from the Improving Palliative Care in the ICU Project Advisory Board and the Center to Advance Palliative Care. *Crit Care Med*. 2015;**43**:1964–77.

Holloway RG, Arnold RM, Creutzfeldt CJ, et al. Palliative and end-of-life care in stroke: A statement for healthcare professionals from the American Heart Association/ American Stroke Association. *Stroke*. 2014;**45**:1887–1916.

Liu Y, Kline D, Aerts S, et al. Inpatient palliative care for neurological disorders: Lessons from a large retrospective series. *J Palliat Med*. 2017;**20**:59–64.

Qaseem A, Snow V, Shekelle P, et al., Clinical Efficacy Assessment Subcommittee of the American College of Physicians. Evidence-based interventions to improve the palliative care of pain, dyspnea, and depression at the end of life: A clinical practice guideline from the American College of Physicians. *Ann Intern Med*. 2008;**148**:141–6.

Quill CM, Quill TE. Palliative use of noninvasive ventilation: Navigating murky waters. *J Palliat Med*. 2014;**17**:657–61.

Stroke and End-Stage Heart Failure

Lauren K. Ng

Clinical History

A 57-year-old man with a history of hypertension, coronary artery disease, diabetes, and hyperlipidemia presented with right-sided weakness. His National Institute of Health Stroke Scale was 24 on arrival to the emergency department, and IV tissue plasminogen activator (tPA) was given 115 minutes after he was last seen normal. A CT angiogram and perfusion of the brain was done, which revealed a left middle cerebral artery M1 segment occlusion with areas of ischemia and penumbra. He was taken to interventional radiology, where a mechanical thrombectomy was performed.

He was also in acute systolic heart failure on admission with acute on chronic kidney injury, bilateral pleural effusions, and pulmonary edema with an ejection fraction of 20–25 percent. He was started on low-dose dobutamine and bilateral pleural pigtail catheters were placed to drain the effusions. An echocardiogram also revealed a left ventricular thrombus and he was started on a heparin drip.

The patient was extubated and weaned off inotropes and started on Lasix, metoprolol, and spironolactone. His neurologic exam had improved and he was attempting to speak and interact, but he remained paralyzed on the right side. He was transferred to the floor while awaiting rehabilitation placement, but he returned to the intensive care unit (ICU) 13 days later in cardiogenic shock and acute respiratory failure requiring intubation, inotropes, and vasopressors.

He was eventually extubated and weaned off inotropes and vasopressors, but had complications of acute kidney injury requiring hemodialysis and acute pancreatitis. On hospital day 29, the patient went into pulseless electrical activity (PEA) arrest with return of spontaneous circulation due to cardiogenic shock. Given his multiple medical comorbidities, his worsened neurologic examination, and end organ failure, palliative care was consulted to assist with end-of-life discussions.

Examination

The patient is intubated and his Glasgow Coma Score is 9T. His eyes were open spontaneously and he would withdraw to noxious stimuli in the left arm and leg, but he could not follow commands.

Palliative Domains of Care

Spiritual Aspects of Care

Respecting the patient's Buddhist faith. The patient was a devout Buddhist, and it was important to incorporate his faith and beliefs into his end-of-life care.

Cultural Aspects of Care

Language barriers with the family. The patient and his wife are originally from Cambodia and have two adult children. As the wife's English was poor, a Cambodian interpreter was requested to assist with the family meeting to eliminate any language barriers.

Palliative Care Discussion

The palliative care discussion focused on discussing the patient's poor prognosis due to multiple organ system failure and progressive neurological decline in the setting of multiple medical complications. The patient's wife and daughter expressed that they would not want him to suffer and they were open to the possibility of withdrawing life-prolonging interventions such as dialysis, vasopressors, and mechanical ventilation. His wife expressed a strong desire for the patient to be able to touch his beloved dog again and she also wanted their son, who lived in Seattle, to be present prior to the withdrawal of life support. It was also important for them to incorporate their Buddhist faith and she requested that their monk perform a customary ceremony before he died.

Hospital Course

The patient was deemed too unstable to transfer to hospice extubated in order to see his dog. Thus, on hospital day 33, after the patient's son arrived, the patient was transferred out of the ICU on the ventilator to a different floor, where the family was able to bring their dog for him to touch prior to the removal of life support. His entire family and members of the Cambodian community were present to say their goodbyes. The patient's Buddhist monk performed the ceremony, and in the presence of his family and his dog, the patient was compassionately weaned from the ventilator and he died several hours later.

General Remarks

This patient presented with multiple comorbidities and subsequently declined over the course of his hospital stay due to multiple in-hospital complications of his chronic illnesses. It was important to include all members of his family in the discussion and to eliminate any language barrier that may have been present by having an appropriate interpreter involved. The family was receptive and reasonable in pursuing withdrawal of life-sustaining care in this situation. It was important to them that we address their goals of having him touch his dog again and of having the Buddhist monk perform a ceremony, which we were able to accomplish.

Suggested Reading

Frontera JA, Curtis JR, Nelson JE et al. Integrating palliative care into the care of the neurocritically ill patients: A report from the Improving Palliative Care in the ICU Project Advisory Board and the Center to Advance Palliative Care. *Crit Care Med* 2015;**43**:1964–77.

Khosla A, Washington KT, Shaunfield S, Slakson R. Communication challenges and strategies of U.S. health professionals caring for seriously ill South Asian patients and their families. *J Palliat Med.* 2017; ahead of print.

Stroke and Decompressive Hemicraniectomy in a Young Patient

Lauren K. Ng

Clinical History

A right-handed 45-year-old woman with a history of hypertension presented with new left hemiplegia and facial droop. In the emergency department, she had a National Institute of Health Stroke Scale (NIHSS) score of 19 and was given IV tissue plasminogen activator (TPA) within 90 minutes of symptom onset. A CT angiogram and perfusion of the head and neck was performed that revealed a proximal right middle cerebral artery (MCA) stenosis with distal embolus with a large matched perfusion defect, suggesting infarction with a smaller area of surrounding penumbra. Given her young age and some areas of ischemia, the patient was taken for mechanical thrombectomy and intubated for airway protection.

The next day, a repeat CT scan of the brain was performed that showed evolving ischemic changes and the development of cerebral edema with midline shift (Figure 14.1). Given the patient's young age and cerebral edema at post-stroke day 1,

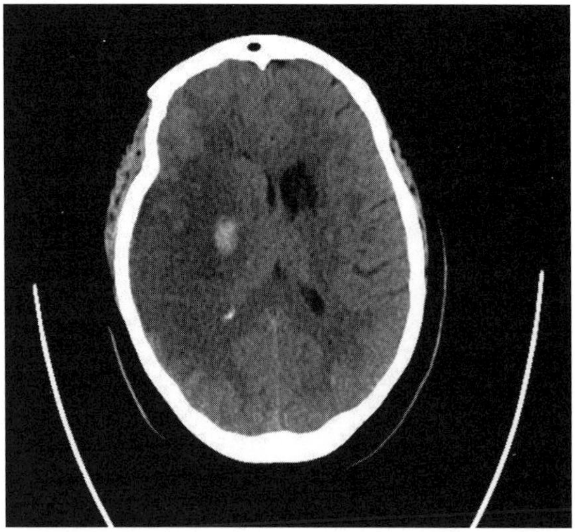

Figure 14.1 Axial non-contrast head CT reveals a right middle cerebral artery stroke with edema, midline shift, and hemorrhagic conversion

a discussion was held with her husband regarding a decompressive hemicraniectomy, given the possibility of worsened, life-threatening cerebral edema over the next 24 hours. It was explained that the procedure would be life-saving, but that it would not recover neurologic function already compromised by the stroke. The husband decided to proceed with a hemicraniectomy.

The next day, the patient's neurologic exam worsened and a repeat CT head revealed a new right cerebellar stroke, left MCA stroke, and enlargement of her right MCA stroke. Given her worsened exam and new strokes, the ICU team met with her husband to discuss her likely neurologic deficits and probable functional outcome. He was informed that at best she may be able to communicate, but that she would be wheelchair bound and paralyzed on the left, requiring 24-hour care. Palliative care was consulted to address goals of care, specifically tracheostomy and gastrostomy tube (PEG) placement if she were unable to be weaned off the ventilator in the setting of severe disability.

Examination

She was intubated and off sedation. Her Glasgow Coma Scale was 8T. She opened her eyes to pain and she was not following commands. She moved her right arm and leg spontaneously, but non-purposefully. Her left arm had extensor posturing with noxious stimuli and her left leg was plegic.

Palliative Domains of Care

Structure and Processes of Care

Prognosis and goals of care. In this scenario, the patient's prognosis was not clear, therefore making the goals of care decision difficult for the family. They knew that she would not want to be sustained on life support if she had impaired cognition and had no degree of independence. However, the medical team had difficulty providing a concrete long-term prognosis given the patient's young age with a non-dominant hemisphere stroke.

Social Aspects of Care

Family support. The family required a significant amount of emotional support as they wrestled with their decision about tracheostomy and PEG tube placement. They were unable to commit to a course of action and they relied heavily on the palliative care team for support and validation.

Palliative Care Discussion

Her family knew her well, but they had never had a discussion regarding what she deemed as an acceptable quality of life. She had not completed an advance directive, but they knew that she would not want to remain on life-sustaining therapies if there was no chance of a reasonable recovery. Discussions with the family centered on the patient's prognosis and functional deficits and their understanding of what they thought would be acceptable to her. Based on what they knew about her values, they noted that an acceptable quality of life would include the ability to communicate, having her cognition intact, and having some degree of independence.

In the absence of a designated health care surrogate, her husband was identified as her health care proxy, according to the state law. The patient's adult children were also heavily involved in the decision-making process.

Despite very detailed conversations prior to her surgery about the life-saving nature of the procedure and that her neurological deficits would not be reversed, her family explained that they remained hopeful that the hemicraniectomy would yield a good outcome. They were conflicted about their decision regarding further life-sustaining treatments, given her marginal neurologic exam and unknown long-term trajectory; however, they decided to proceed with tracheostomy and PEG tube to allow her additional time to recover.

In meeting with the family, the palliative care team learned that this was a very close-knit family. The patient and her husband had known each other for 25 years, were married for 15 years, and had three adult children. Their children all lived at home, they ate dinner each night together as a family, and the patient and her husband had date night each Saturday. They were co-dependent on each other and neither her husband nor her children could imagine a life without her. They were also a family with a strong faith in God and they fervently prayed for her recovery and healing. Understanding these details of her social situation provided a better understanding for the medical team about factors that may influence her family's decision-making.

Hospital Course

The patient received a tracheostomy and PEG, but did not improve neurologically. She developed ICU delirium and pneumonia and required prolonged ventilation. She was eventually transferred out of the ICU to the progressive care unit (PCU) while awaiting long-term acute care placement. She was on aspirin and warfarin with a heparin bridge for secondary stroke prevention for a hypercoagulable state. On day 25 of her hospital stay, the family noted fullness at her surgical site; repeat CT head imaging revealed a large subdural hematoma and midline shift (Figure 14.2). She was transferred back to the ICU and she continued to decline neurologically. Based on her poor prognosis and an unreasonable expectation for recovery to a functional status that would be acceptable to her, her family opted not to pursue additional surgical options, and the patient progressed to brain death.

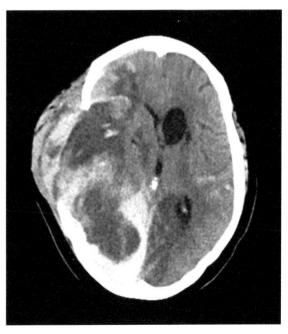

Figure 14.2 Axial non-contrast head CT after a decompressive hemicraniectomy. A right subdural hematoma is present.

General Remarks

Unfortunately in this situation, the patient had not designated a health care surrogate and she had not spoken to her family in advance about her preferences for end-of-life care. In addition, the family had false expectations and a poor understanding from the beginning about her recovery potential after surgery, and they remained conflicted about their decisions due to an unknown long-term prognosis.

Outcome prediction in the neuro-critical care unit is difficult. In addition, prognosis could not be accurately predicted in the first day after the stroke when the decision for surgery needed to be made. Physicians have been cautioned against addressing end-of-life issues in the neuro-critical care unit too early in the hospital course as it could lead to a self-fulfilling prophecy. Multiple discussions with the family helped build rapport and trust so when the patient developed a catastrophic hemorrhage, the family felt comfortable not pursuing additional aggressive treatment and allowing natural death.

Suggested Reading

Cai X, Robinson J, Muehlschlegel S et al. Patient preferences and surrogate decision making in neuroscience intensive care units. *Neurocrit Care*. 2015;**23**: 131–41.

Frontera JA, Curtis JR, Nelson JE, et al. Integrating palliative care into the care of neurocritically ill patients: A report from the Improving Palliative Care in the ICU Project Advisory Board and the Center to Advance Palliative Care. *Critical care medicine*. 2015;**43**(9): 1964–77.

Hofmeijer J, Kappelle LJ, Algra A, Amelink GJ, van Gijn J, van der Worp B, et al. Surgical decompression for space-occupying cerebral infarction (the Hemicraniectomy after Middle Cerebral Artery Infarction with Life-Threatening Edema Trial [HAMLET]): A multicentre, open, randomised trial. *Lancet Neurol*. 2009;**8**(4): 326–33.

Rubin M, Bonomo J, Hemphill JC. Intersection of prognosis and palliation in neurocritical care. *Curr Opin Crit Care*. 2017;**23**:134–9.

Surrogate Decision-Making after a Malignant MCA Ischemic Stroke

Breana L. Taylor and Claire J. Creutzfeldt

Clinical History

A 73-year-old right-handed man with a medical history significant for hypertension, end-stage renal disease status post renal transplant, and paroxysmal atrial fibrillation was brought into the emergency department by his daughter after being found on the floor of his apartment with right hemiplegia and aphasia. He had been last seen normal 12 hours prior to presentation. His initial National Institute of Health Stroke Scale (NIHSS) score was 27. A non-contrast head CT showed no acute hemorrhage, but did show early ischemia involving a large portion of the left middle cerebral artery (MCA) territory. The CT angiogram showed an occlusion of the proximal left M1 branch of the MCA. He was outside the time window and therefore not a candidate for acute interventions, including intravenous tissue plasminogen activator (t-PA) administration or mechanical thrombectomy. He became less responsive over the course of the day and an MRI of his brain showed restricted diffusion in the entire left MCA distribution with early signs of mass effect (Figures 15.1 and 15.2). A decision had to be made about whether to proceed with a decompressive hemicraniectomy.

Evidence suggests malignant MCA stroke in older patients has a 70 percent six-month mortality when treated with medical therapy alone, versus 30 percent if patients receive early surgical management. Survival without dependence is rare in both groups [1]. Early surgery suggests not waiting until clinical signs of active herniation are apparent.

Examination

He was afebrile, hypertensive 210/112, and tachycardic with an irregularly irregular rhythm (110). He was drowsy but easily arousable to tactile stimuli. He was mute and unable to follow any commands. He had a left gaze preference, right hemiplegia, and dense sensory loss on the right.

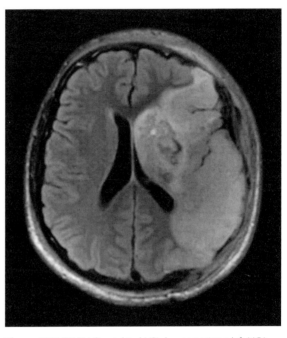

Figure 15.1 T2 FLAIR weighted MRI demonstrating a left MCA distribution ischemic infarct with edema and mass effect

Palliative Domain of Care

Structure and Process of Care – Effective communication in the acute setting and goal concordant care

Background and social context: Despite his history of chronic medical conditions, the patient had been doing well in the recent past. His daughter described him as vibrant and fun loving. He had been a "fighter" for most of his life, but after his wife died one year prior, he seemed more withdrawn, less willing to take his medications or visit his doctors regularly. He was still living independently, and he enjoyed monthly fishing trips with his brother and playing with his five-year-old grandson daily.

He had not completed any formal advance directives, nor had any specific conversations with his

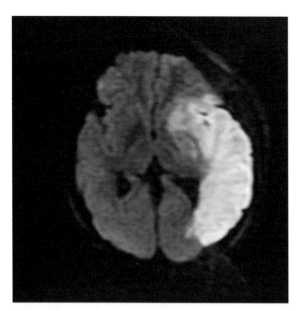

Figure 15.2 MRI DWI sequence demonstrating a large left MCA distribution ischemic infarct

daughter about life-sustaining measures. His daughter acknowledged that his quality of life had suffered greatly after his wife died, and she wondered if life after a malignant dominant hemisphere MCA stroke would be acceptable to her father.

Palliative Care Discussion

The patient's daughter arrived to the emergency department alone. When asked if there was anyone else she would like to include in the discussion, she stated that the patient had three younger siblings who did not live locally, but with whom he had maintained regular contact. She did not have their phone numbers at the time of the discussion.

Family understanding and perspective of illness: The patient's daughter understood that he had suffered a severe stroke, which was affecting his ability to speak and to move his right side. She had hoped that he would improve back to his independent baseline, but she was starting to recognize the severity of his stroke and the high probability of prolonged, likely permanent, severe disability.

Acceptable quality of life: The patient's daughter was unsure if her father would want to live if he were dependent on other people. This was especially true in light of his recent aversion to the health care system.

She understood that the decision for surgery had to be made quickly to give him the best chance at

survival. Although she was his legal next of kin, she felt uncomfortable making such a big decision on her own. She therefore preferred that the patient be full code and that aggressive medical therapy be continued until she could confer with the patient's siblings.

Hospital Course

He was intubated in the emergency department for an inability to protect his airway. He was started on a hypertonic saline drip and admitted to the neurologic intensive care unit. His brainstem reflexes were all intact at the time of admission. After 16 hours, he began to require significant increases of his nicardipine drip. He was also noted to have asymmetric pupils and absent corneal reflexes bilaterally. His daughter had been unable to reach all of the patient's siblings by this point, but she had talked to his youngest sister. Together, they decided that he would be unhappy with the degree of residual disability if he were to survive the acute phase of his stroke. Trying to use substituted judgment, they felt that a decompressive hemicraniectomy would not align with the goals of care. Therefore, he was transitioned to comfort measures only and he was compassionately extubated. He died a few hours later.

General Remarks

In the setting of an acute stroke, neurologists frequently find themselves in the situation where treatment decisions require balancing patient preferences with the anticipated burden or benefit of the treatment [2]. Given the acute and unexpected nature of stroke, family members are often left having to make inferences about what their loved one would have wanted were they able to participate in these conversations. While experiencing acute loss, family members should not be asked to make these decisions on their own. Establishing trust with the patient's family is a crucial early step in caring for the patient with sudden onset, life-changing illness. Trust-building includes honest, clear, and direct communication regarding the severity of the situation, without overwhelming the family with medical jargon, and empathic listening. These crucial conversations are challenging in the chaotic environment that is created by the acute injury and the "time is brain" imperative in the emergency room and characterized by substantial uncertainty, stress, and grief for patients, family members, and care providers [3].

The first meeting with the family should focus on developing a trusting relationship. Communication should always start with introductions. The second step is to elicit the family's current understanding of the situation. Asking the family what they have heard not only avoids redundancy but more importantly helps providers sense the family's level of understanding, their illness perspective, and their coping mechanisms. Next, the provider provides an accurate representation of the situation, using language the family can understand and limiting the description to key points. At this point, the provider should pause. This pause may feel awkward, but it is important for eliciting and tending to emotions and concerns of the family. Without addressing these things early on in the conversation, it may be difficult for the family to focus on the decision-making aspects of the discussion. This is a good time to try to elicit the patient's values, who they are, what brings their life meaning, and what they might consider an acceptable quality of life. Establishing what is important to the patient will help the family and medical providers make decisions that are in line with the patient's prior stated or inferred values and provide goal-concordant care. The last part of the conversation includes a brief discussion of the immediate next steps and any major procedures that may be indicated in the short term. The appropriateness of any urgent interventions should be addressed with a specific focus on whether they are in line with the patient's values. Acknowledge that further discussions may be indicated depending on the clinical course. The family should be informed of ways to communicate with members of the medical team should additional questions or concerns arise and they should be checked in with frequently.

In this particular situation, it was important for the medical team to support and reassure the patient's daughter, who was struggling with feeling that she was making a decision to end her father's life. Reframing this thought by reviewing the patient's values and preferences about other issues helped her realize that goal-concordant care for her father involved making him comfortable through this situation rather than pursuing aggressive surgical intervention [4].

Suggested Reading

1. Juttler E, Unterberg A, Woitzik J, et al. Hemicraniectomy in older patients with extensive middle-cerebral-artery stroke. *N Engl J Med.* 2014;**370**(12):1091–1100.

2. Creutzfeldt CJ, Longstreth WT, Holloway RG. Predicting decline and survival in severe acute brain injury: The fourth trajectory. *BMJ.* 2015;**351**:h3904.

3. Creutzfeldt CJ, Holloway RG, Curtis JR. Palliative care: A core competency for stroke neurologists. *Stroke.* 2015;**46**(9):2714–19.

4. Quill TE, Holloway RG. Evidence, preferences, recommendations – finding the right balance in patient care. *N Engl J Med.* 2012;**366**(18):1653–5.

16 A Time-Limited Trial in a Case of a Basilar Artery Occlusion

Breana L. Taylor and Claire J. Creutzfeldt

Clinical History

A 41-year-old right-handed woman with no known medical history developed sudden-onset, left neck pain, headache, vertigo, nausea, and vomiting while teaching her third grade class. Her aide called 911 and paramedics arrived within 10 minutes. She was unresponsive upon their assessment and was intubated on the scene. She was brought to the emergency department, a stroke code was called, and she was rushed directly to the CT scanner. A non-contrast CT scan showed no acute hemorrhage or early ischemic changes, but suggested a hyperdense basilar artery. A CT angiogram confirmed a basilar artery occlusion and left vertebral artery irregularity concerning for dissection. The initial National Institute of Health Stroke Scale (NIHSS) score was 28. Tissue plasminogen activator (t-PA) was administered 85 minutes after symptom onset. She was taken to the angiography suite, where mechanical thrombectomy was performed, and a large clot was removed from the basilar artery.

She had no immediate complications from intravenous (t-PA) or the procedure and she was admitted to the neurologic intensive care unit. At 24 hours post t-PA and thrombectomy the patient remained comatose.

An MRI of her brain showed a large area of restricted diffusion in her bilateral pons, as well as scattered punctate infarcts of the bilateral cerebellar hemispheres with relative sparing of the upper midbrain.

Examination

On hospital day 12, she was hypertensive (160/95), but other vital signs were within normal limits. She had passed several spontaneous breathing trials, but she failed a trial of extubation and she therefore remained intubated for airway protection. She rarely opened her eyes spontaneously. She had pinpoint pupils. Horizontal vestibular ocular reflex was absent, but vertical eye movements were present upon passive head flexion and extension. She had extensor (decerebrate) posturing of her extremities to central pain, and her right lower extremity exhibited triple flexion to peripheral pain.

Palliative Domain of Care

Ethical and Legal Aspects of Care – Decision-making about tracheostomy, enteral feeding options, and time-limited trials

Background and social context: The patient was a young elementary school teacher who lived with her husband and two children, ages five and eight. She was considered outgoing by most of her friends, and had recently been spending her weekends organizing a party for her parents' fiftieth wedding anniversary. She had no prior medical problems and had never had any conversations with her husband or her parents about her preferences regarding artificial nutrition or prolonged life-sustaining measures. Both her husband and parents felt that she would not want to live forever in a vegetative state, but given that she was otherwise healthy and had two young children, they hoped that she would make improvements over time.

The patient was nearing the two-week mark of hospitalization and had not made any significant clinical improvements. While her prognosis remained uncertain, her clinical picture over the first 12 days and the location of her infarct suggested that she would require prolonged artificial life support, including a tracheostomy and percutaneous gastrostomy tube (PEG).

Palliative Care Discussion

Family understanding and perspective of illness: The family all agreed that she would want to be given every possible chance for recovery because of her two young children. They expressed frustration that she had not made any prominent improvements over the 12 days since her admission. They understood that although they hoped that she would ultimately return to being independent, this was unlikely going to be an attainable goal.

Acceptable quality of life: Her family and spending time with her loved ones gave this patient's life meaning and purpose. Her family believed that if she could still interact with them in some meaningful way, this would be an acceptable outcome to her.

The indications for tracheostomy tube and PEG tube placement were reviewed. Although her mother recognized the need to transition from oral intubation to the tracheostomy tube, she had concerns about her daughter needing permanent artificial nutrition. She wanted the medical providers to provide her with an estimate of the chances that her daughter would ever "wake up." The possibility of recovery to a state of locked-in syndrome was discussed. Although the patient had not exhibited the ability to reliably communicate up to this point, the speech therapist was hopeful that the patient would be able to eventually participate in some form of communication.

Given her young age and her presumed goals and values, the lack of cortical involvement on her MRI, and the possibility of awakening, the family decided to move forward with tracheostomy and PEG tube placement. Given that greatest recovery after stroke occurs in the first three to six months, the family planned to reassess the her progress with her vascular neurologist after three months. If she were not improving substantially and showing an ability to reliably communicate with her family, withdrawal of artificial life support and transition to comfort measures only could be discussed.

Hospital Course

Tracheostomy tube and PEG tube were successfully placed on hospital day 14. She was quickly weaned off of mechanical ventilation by hospital day 15.

On hospital day 17 she was noted to be more consistently following commands to open or close her eyes. She continued to be unable to move her lower face or any of her extremities spontaneously.

On hospital day 18 she was noted by speech therapy to answer 70 percent of yes/no egocentric questions correctly with blinking, but only 50 percent of non-egocentric questions correctly.

On hospital day 23 she was discharged to a skilled nursing facility to continue to work with speech, physical, and occupational therapy.

General Remarks

Prognostication in the previously healthy, young stroke patient can be very challenging [1]. Despite our best efforts, there are few reliable measures to predict the degree to which an individual patient will improve after their stroke, or the degree to which they might adjust to their deficits. The use of time-limited trials can be helpful in the setting of substantial uncertainty. Time-limited trials are an agreement between clinicians and a patient/family to use certain medical therapies over a defined period of time to see if the patient improves or deteriorates according to agreed-on clinical outcomes [2]. A time-limited trial provides clinicians more data points upon which to base neuro-prognostic statements and gives families more time to understand benefits and burdens of therapy and to work through grief. When discussing a time-limited trial with family members, it is important that the duration of the trial, the frequency of check-ins, and the possible steps taken following those are agreed on up front. Assuring the family that they are not being abandoned is crucial. Ideally, the same provider should follow the patient longitudinally after discharge from the hospital in order to facilitate trust building in the outpatient setting and to help the family arrive at what may be a difficult decision once the time limited trial is complete.

Basilar artery occlusion and the possibility of locked-in syndrome presented an interesting additional challenge to neuro-prognostication in this case. Several studies have shown that many people with chronic locked-in syndrome report having a satisfactory quality of life on self-assessment [3]. An aggressive attempt to work with these patients in an effort to develop communication strategies is important. They may even be able to eventually participate in ongoing discussions about their own goals of care.

Suggested Reading

1. Creutzfeldt CJ, Holloway RG. Treatment decisions after severe stroke: Uncertainty and biases. *Stroke*. 2012;**43**(12):3405–8.

2. Quill TE, Holloway R. Time-limited trials near the end of life. *JAMA*. 2011;**306**(13):1483–4.

3. Bruno MA, Bernheim JL, Ledoux D, Pellas F, Demertzi A, Laureys S. A survey on self-assessed well-being in a cohort of chronic locked-in syndrome patients: Happy majority, miserable minority. *BMJ Open*. 2011;**1**(1):e000039.

"Mom Never Wanted a Feeding Tube"

Maisha T. Robinson

Clinical History

A 91-year-old woman with a history of hypertension, diabetes, atrial fibrillation, falls, and mild dementia presented with aphasia and right hemiparesis. Upon evaluation in the emergency department, she had a National Institute of Health Stroke Scale Score (NIHSS) of 15. A non-contrast head CT showed early ischemic changes in the posterior left middle cerebral artery territory (Figure 17.1). She received 0.9 mg/kg of intravenous recombinant tissue plasminogen activator (rt-PA) 105 minutes after her symptoms began.

Seven hours later, she became agitated and her NIHSS worsened to 24. A non-contrast head CT demonstrated a right temporal hematoma, concerning for an amyloid angiopathy-related hemorrhage (Figure 17.2). Her tPA coagulopathy was reversed with cryoprecipitate, platelets, and fresh frozen plasma.

On day 3 of her hospitalization, she was alert enough to attempt a swallow evaluation, which demonstrated severe oral and pharyngeal dysphagia.

Examination

She was afebrile, tachycardic (117 beats per minute), and hypertensive (161/99 mmHg). She was awake and alert. She was globally aphasic with unintelligible

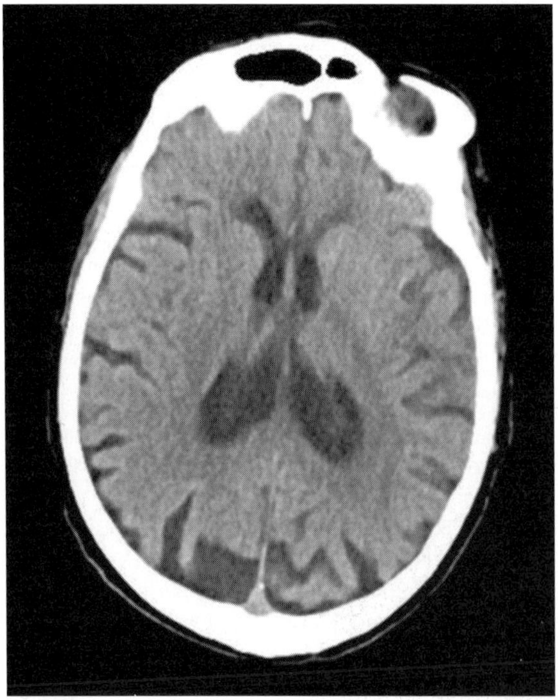

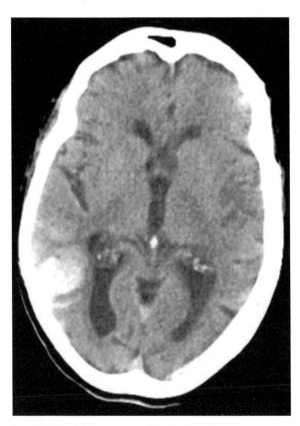

Figure 17.1 Axial non-contrast head CT showing an acute infarct in the left posterior middle cerebral artery territory

Figure 17.2 Axial non-contrast head CT showing an intraparenchymal hemorrhage in the right posterior temporal lobe

verbal output, marked dysarthria, a left gaze preference, and right hemiplegia.

Palliative Domain of Care

Ethical and Legal Aspects of Care – Decision-making about enteral feeding options

The patient had not completed an advance directive, but she had designated one of her children as her health care surrogate. She had told her children in prior discussions that she never wanted a feeding tube and that she never wanted to be in a nursing facility, as she identified those care measures with impending death. She also stated that she did not want to be resuscitated.

Her children were unsure if temporary feeding options would be acceptable to their mother. They attempted to engage her in the conversation, but as a result of her aphasia, it was difficult for them to discern her thoughts about the situation. Her children had differing opinions regarding whether a feeding tube should be placed.

Palliative Care Discussion

The patient's prior, stated wishes for no feeding tube suggested that her preference was for less aggressive measures in the setting of a serious medical condition. However, in the absence of an advance directive, the decision regarding life-sustaining measures was left to her designated health care surrogate.

The discussion with her family included an understanding of her premorbid functioning. Prior to her hospitalization, she had been living with one of her children for the past several years. She was able to manage the majority of her activities of daily living independently, including bathing, dressing, feeding, and toileting. Given her dementia, which primarily manifested as short-term memory loss and paranoia, her children assisted her with medication management and with meal preparation. She ambulated with a gait aid and she had approximately one fall a year without serious injuries. Her family thought that she enjoyed her quality of life.

Given the findings on her initial head CT scan, her older age, in-hospital decline, severe neurologic deficits, and poor rehabilitation potential, her chance for a return to her baseline function was low [1, 2].

Her children were unsure what decision their mother would make under these circumstances and they were unable to reach a consensus. Therefore, they decided to proceed with a percutaneous gastrostomy tube with the hope that it would provide her with nutrition and that it would allow for ease of medication administration. They hoped that the tube would be temporary. The alternative option of transitioning the patient's care to comfort was also discussed.

Hospital Course

On day 6 of her hospitalization, she acutely developed tachypnea, tachycardia, and dyspnea. A CT angiogram of the chest demonstrated a nonocclusive left lower lobe subsegmental pulmonary embolism and bilateral pleural effusions. In discussion with the neurology team, her children elected not to pursue anticoagulation due to the risk of further intraparenchymal hemorrhage.

On day 7 of her hospitalization, a percutaneous gastrostomy tube was placed. After the tube was placed, the patient pulled it out; it was reinserted, and she subsequently required wrist restraints. Over the next several hours, she became increasingly more uncomfortable and agitated. A non-contrast head CT revealed interval progression of the right posterior temporal intraparenchymal hemorrhage.

On day 8 of her hospitalization, extremity ultrasounds revealed a nonocclusive deep vein thrombosis in the right femoral vein and an occlusive deep vein thrombosis in the right brachial vein. She required low-dose opioids and benzodiazepines for agitation, dyspnea, and pleuritic chest pain.

The palliative care team met with her family routinely to review the daily medical events, provide support for her children, and continue discussions regarding goals of care. With each new setback, her children came closer to reaching a consensus regarding the next best step for their mother. They ultimately decided that their mother's current quality of life – and her future quality of life – would not have been acceptable to her. Based on their desire to grant her peace and comfort, hospice was consulted.

General Remarks

In the absence of clear, documented preferences for end-of-life care, a designated health care surrogate or a health care proxy is tasked with the responsibility of guiding the complex decisions for life-prolonging and end-of-life care if the patient lacks the capacity to make those decisions. In this case, the patient had designated one of her children as her health care surrogate. Although the surrogate and her siblings had discussions with their mother prior to the hospitalization, they were unsure as to what decision to make regarding enteral feeding options in this particular situation. They were hopeful that she could recover from her neurologic and medical conditions and they were therefore unsure if her previously expressed wishes applied in this instance.

It can be challenging to determine the level of care intensity that a person would want if specific conversations had not been held prior to a stroke. Palliative medicine teams may be consulted to assist with clarifying goals of care and to discuss the options regarding treatment preferences. Stroke patients often have fewer traditional symptoms as compared to a general population of palliative care patients. Conversations with stroke patients and their caregivers often center on issues related to life-prolonging care, such as artificial nutrition and hydration [3].

Throughout her hospitalization, her medical condition progressively declined and her clinical course led to a series of discussions regarding her care. Not uncommonly, as the situation changes, goals of care need to be readdressed, as they were with this patient. With the assistance of the medical team, her family realized that she was not going to improve to her prior level of functioning, which is what she would have deemed an acceptable quality of life.

Early discussions with the patient's family included the option of comfort care and hospice. When they were ready to transition the patient's care to hospice, comfort measures were initiated. She died peacefully several hours later surrounded by her family.

Suggested Reading

1. Adams HP Jr., Davis PH, Leira EC, et al. Baseline NIH Stroke Scale score strongly predicts outcome after stroke: A report of the Trial of Org 10172 in Acute Stroke Treatment (TOAST). *Neurology*. 1999; 53:126.

2. Kammersgaard LP, Jørgensen HS, Reith J, et al. Short- and long-term prognosis for very old stroke patients. *The Copenhagen Stroke Study. Age Ageing* 2004;**33**:149.

3. Holloway RG, Ladwig S, Robb J, Kelly A, Nielsen E, Quill TE. Palliative care consultations in hospitalized stroke patients. *J Palliat Med.* 2010 Apr;**13**(4):407–12.

4. Holloway RG, Arnold RM, Creutzfeldt CJ, Lewis EF, Lutz BJ, McCann RM, Rabinstein AA, Saposnik G, Sheth KN, Zahuranec DB, Zipfel GJ, Zorowitz RD. Palliative and end-of-life care in stroke: A statement for healthcare professionals from the American Heart Association/American Stroke Association. *Stroke.* 2014 Jun;**45**(6):1887–916.

5. Creutzfeldt CJ, Holloway RG. Treatment decisions after severe stroke: Uncertainty and biases. *Stroke.* 2012 Dec;**43**(12):3405–8.

Chapter

18 Painfully Cold, Numb, and Weak
Clinical Characteristics and Management of Central Post-stroke Pain

Neha M. Kramer

Clinical History

MO is a 61-year-old woman with a history of refractory hypertension, hyperlipidemia, obstructive sleep apnea, and obesity, who experienced sudden-onset left hemiparesis and weakness, preceded by paresthesias of the left arm while at home. She presented to the emergency department, where her systolic blood pressure was elevated to 240 mmHg. A head CT showed a right thalamic intracerebral hemorrhage (ICH) extending into the posterior limb of the internal capsule measuring 2.0 x 1.5 x 2.4 cm. The hematoma was surrounded by a thin rim of edema, with minimal mass effect on the right lateral ventricle, without midline shift or intraventricular hemorrhage (Figure 18.1). ICH score was 0. National Institute of Health Stroke Scale (NIHSS) score was 11.

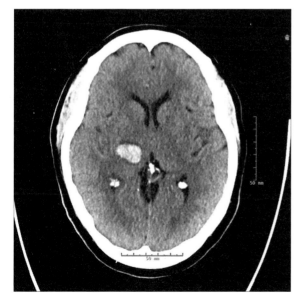

Figure 18.1 Axial non-contrast head CT shows an acute hematoma in the right thalamocapsular region with minimal compression of the right lateral ventricle

Examination

Her exam on admission was notable for severe left hemiparesis of the face, arm, and leg, with mild left hemi-sensory loss to pinprick and mild dysarthria. She was awake, alert, and fully oriented. There was no evidence of aphasia.

Clinical Course

The etiology of the ICH was determined to be hypertensive. Her hypertension was initially managed with IV antihypertensive agents, with eventual transition to her home oral regimen consisting of five medications. Over the following days, she regained some strength and sensation of her left hemi-body. NIHSS improved to 8. On the third day of admission, she developed aching pain in the left leg, with superimposed intermittent shooting pain and painfully cold sensations. A few days later she developed stabbing pain on the left side of her face and aching left shoulder pain. Her pain was not associated with movement. An x-ray of the left shoulder was unremarkable. She was diagnosed with thalamic central post-stroke syndrome. Her pain improved with the initiation and titration of gabapentin to 300 mg three times daily. She was initially discharged to acute rehabilitation, then home seven weeks later. Her Modified Rankin Scale (MRS) at the time of discharge home was 4.

At MO's three-month follow-up visit, she reported moderate improvement in strength, though she still required assistance with activities of daily living. The pain in the left hemi-body had become excruciating; she had developed sensitivity to light touch, which limited her ability to use this arm. Gabapentin was further increased to 600 mg three times daily. She was also started on amitriptyline for low mood related to limited independence and unrelenting pain.

At MO's three-year follow-up visit, her pain persisted, though was well controlled on gabapentin 600 mg three times daily. She was able to perform most activities of daily living independently. Her neurological exam was notable for mild left upper and lower extremity weakness, mild decreased sensation to pinprick in the left hemi-body, and dysesthesia to cold temperature in the left arm and face. NIHSS was 4 and MRS was 3.

Domain of Palliative Care

Physical Aspects of Care – Central post-stroke pain

A core principle of palliative care is symptom management, including pain. Pain is categorized as either neuropathic pain or nociceptive pain, which is further divided into somatic and visceral types of pain. Palliative care evaluations involve detailed pain assessments, including the characteristics of the pain, exacerbating or alleviating factors, location and severity of the pain, limitations secondary to pain, and associated symptoms. Management plans may include pharmacologic and non-pharmacologic treatment options.

Palliative Care Discussion

Stroke is the leading cause of disability and one of the most common causes of death in the United States. In the literature, there is minimal focus on supportive symptom management for stroke survivors, yet attention to disabling symptoms can significantly improve quality of life and is often what matters most to stroke patients and their families.

Various studies show 11–55 percent of stroke survivors suffer from chronic pain as a consequence of stroke [1]. The most common post-stroke pain syndromes are hemiplegic shoulder pain (20 percent), central post-stroke pain (CPSP) (10 percent), persistent headache (10 percent), and spasticity (7 percent) [1]. Patients may have more than one type of post-stroke pain. Chronic pain after stroke has been shown to reduce quality of life and impede rehabilitation, as well as negatively impact sleep, mood, and overall function [2].

CPSP is a neuropathic pain syndrome that can occur when a stroke lesion disrupts the central somatosensory system (thalamic ventral posterior nuclei, lateral medulla, or sensory cortex), resulting in spinothalamic or thalamocortical tract dysfunction. Essential to the diagnosis of CPSP, the pain location corresponds to the body region clinically affected by the CNS lesion. Therefore, patients with CPSP from a lateral medullary infarction may experience pain in the ipsilateral face and contralateral body, while those with thalamic infarctions frequently report contralateral hemi-body pain. Interestingly, pain usually does not involve the entire neurologically affected region, just a portion of it. When CPSP results from a thalamic infarct, it historically has been referred to as Dejerine-Roussy Syndrome.

General Remarks

The risk of CPSP is comparable for ischemic and hemorrhagic stroke, and overall incidence is 2–8 percent [3]. Stroke laterality, sex, and age are not consistent risk factors of CPSP [3, 4]. CPSP may occur at stroke onset (as in the case discussed earlier), though more commonly pain arises within weeks to months and sometimes years [3]. Because there is a risk of recurrent strokes in this population, pain onset after six to 12 months should prompt a workup for another cause, such as a new stroke [1]. The delay in temporal onset can make recognition of CPSP challenging, as often these patients have transferred their medical care away from specialty care and back to their primary provider.

If the painful limb has normal pinprick and temperature sensations (indicating intact spinothalamic tract function), the limb pain is unlikely to be related to CPSP and other causes of pain such as nociceptive, psychogenic, or peripheral neuropathic pain should be considered. Unlike hemiplegic shoulder pain or spasticity, the CPSP is not related to movement. Although any pain descriptor can apply, CPSP is often described as electric shocks, burning, painful cold, aching, pressing, stinging, or pins and needles. Allodynia, hyperalgesia, or dysesthesia to touch and cold temperature are common.

When left untreated, the pain from CPSP can be severe, persistent, and intolerable, and in some cases has led to suicide [5]. The treatment of CPSP is challenging and the disappearance of pain is highly unlikely. Several studies for neuropathic pain have consistently shown that combination therapy is more effective than monotherapy [6], yet none of the few randomized controlled trials published for CPSP included combination therapy [1].

Among antidepressants, amitriptyline (75 mg/day) is effective for CPSP and considered a first line treatment [7]. Interestingly, the same medication and

Table 18.1 Treatment of post-stroke pain

Drug	Drug Class	Outcome of Evidence	Effective Dosage
Amitriptyline	Tertiary Amine TCA Antidepressant	Positive	At least 75 mg/day
Duloxetine	SSNRI Antidepressant	None. Effective for other central neuropathic pain states	60 mg/day
Lamotrigine	Anticonvulsant	Positive	200 mg/day
Carbamazepine	Anticonvulsant	Negative	800 mg/day
Gabapentin	Calcium channel a2-d ligands Anticonvulsant	None. Effective for other central neuropathic pain states	At least 1,800 mg/day
Pregabalin	Calcium channel a2-d ligands Anticonvulsant	Mixed	300–600 mg/day
Morphine	Opioid agonist	Mixed. Use in refractory cases	
	Cannabinoids	None. Effective for other central pain states	

dose was not effective for preventing CPSP. Though selective serotonin-norepinephrine reuptake inhibitors (SSNRIs) have not been studied in CPSP, the rationale for considering this class is based on their convincing efficacy for other neuropathic pain syndromes, both central (multiple sclerosis-related pain) and peripheral (painful diabetic neuropathy and chemotherapy-related peripheral neuropathy). Furthermore, SSNRIs may be a safer option than tricyclic antidepressants (TCAs) for patients with cardiac disease. Overall, SSNRIs have been shown to be less effective for neuropathic pain.

For anticonvulsant agents, lamotrigine (200 mg/day) is moderately effective, well tolerated [8], and considered a first-line therapy. Unlike the central neuropathic pain syndrome of trigeminal neuralgia, carbamazepine (800 mg per day) is not effective for CPSP [7]. Gabapentin has not been studied for CPSP, but can be considered a second-line agent based on its efficacy for other central neuropathic pain states (at a dose of at least 1,800 mg/day). Pregabalin (300–600 mg/day) has produced mixed results [9].

Intravenous medications such as lidocaine, propofol, and ketamine are effective for CPSP in the short term; however, their route and side effect profiles render these inappropriate for long-term treatment [10]. Opioids have not been adequately studied for CPSP, are only modestly effective in neuropathic pain states, and therefore only recommended in refractory states. Cannabinoids have not been studied in CPSP, though have shown efficacy for multiple sclerosis-related central pain.

Neuromodulation therapy (e.g., deep brain stimulation, transcranial magnetic stimulation, and motor cortex stimulation) interrupts ascending nociceptive signaling or it activates descending inhibitory pathways, and it has been implemented for intractable cases of CPSP.

Just as in the treatment of other chronic pain states, palliative care principles of promoting a therapeutic relationship, developing mutually agreed-upon meaningful outcomes, and managing outcome expectations are essential when managing CPSP in stroke survivors. Similarly, chronic pain principles of incorporating therapeutic exercise and psychosocial support are also recommended.

Suggested Reading

1. Klit H, Finnerup NB, Jensen TS. Central post-stroke pain: Clinical characteristics, pathophysiology, and management. *Lancet Neurol.* 2009;**8**:857–68.

2. Widar M, Ek AC, Ahlstrom G. Coping with long-term pain after a stroke. *J Pain Symptom Manage.* 2004;**27**: 215–25.

3. Andersen G, Vestergaard K, Ingeman-Nielsen M, Jensen TS. Incidence of central post-stroke pain. *Pain.* 1995;**61**(2):187–93.

4. MacGowan DJ, Janal MN, Clark WC, Wharton RN, Lazar RM, Sacco RL, et al. Central poststroke pain and Wallenberg's lateral medullary infarction: Frequency, character, and determinants in 63 patients. *Neurology.* 1997;**49**(1):120–5.

5. Gonzales GR. Central pain: Diagnosis and treatment strategies. *Neurology.* 1995;**45**:S11–S16.

6. Finnerup NB, Attal N, Haroutounian S, McNicol E, Baron R, Dworkin RH, et al. Pharmacotherapy for neuropathic pain in adults: A systematic review and meta-analysis. *Lancet Neurol.* 2015;**14**(2):162–73.

7. Leijon G, Boivie J. Central post-stroke pain: A controlled trial of amitriptyline and carbamazepine. *Pain.* 1989;**36**(1):27–36.

8. Vestergaard K, Andersen G, Gottrup H, Kristensen BT, Jensen TS. Lamotrigine for central poststroke pain: A randomized controlled trial. *Neurology.* 2001;**56**(2):184–90.

9. Watson JC, Sandroni P. Central neuropathic pain syndromes. *Mayo Clin Proc.* 2016;**91**(3):372–85.

10. Frese A, Husstedt IW, Ringelstein EB, Evers S. Pharmacologic treatment of central post-stroke pain. *Clin J Pain.* 2006;**22**:252–60.

Shared Decision-Making for Stroke Patients
Integrating Patient Values and Life Goals with Best Clinical Evidence to Formulate an Individualized Care Plan

Neha M. Kramer

Clinical History

RT is a 43-year-old woman with a history of profound intellectual disability, hypertension, and poorly controlled diabetes mellitus type 2, who presented to the emergency department with nausea and emesis and was in hyperosmotic hyperglycemic nonketotic state with serum glucose >1,100 mg/dL. A head CT on admission was unremarkable.

Examination

General medical exam was notable for short stature, short neck, and short fourth metacarpals. Neurological exam revealed she was awake and alert; she had baseline paucity of speech and limited vocabulary.

Over the following days, RT became progressively less responsive. By day 6, she opened her eyes briefly to noxious stimulus, did not follow commands, had a left gaze preference, did not blink to threat, had intact brainstem reflexes, and had flexion response to noxious stimuli in all extremities (left more than right). National Institute of Health Stroke Scale (NIHSS) score was 23.

Hospital Course

A repeat CT head revealed multiple large acute ischemic infarcts in the right parietal, right temporal-occipital, and left frontal-parietal lobes without hemorrhagic transformation or mass effect. An MRI brain confirmed multifocal acute ischemic infarctions in the bilateral MCA territories (anterior, posterior, and watershed zones), as well as an acute ischemic infarct in the left medial pons (Figure 19.1). A CT angiography of the head and neck showed complete occlusion just distal to the origin of the left internal carotid artery, severe narrowing of the cervical, petrosal, and cavernous segments of the right ICA with

complete occlusion of the proximal supraclinoid segment of the right ICA, as well as reconstitution of the distal supraclinoid segments of bilateral internal carotid arteries from retrograde flow via posterior communicating arteries. Bilateral middle and anterior cerebral arteries were patent. Moderate stenosis of the V4 segment of the left vertebral artery from atherosclerotic disease was appreciated (Figure 19.2).

Her stroke workup was notable for elevated Rheumatoid Factor (58 IU/mL), ESR (76 mm/hr), and CRP (72.2 mg/L), elevated Hemoglobin A1C (13 percent). A transthoracic echocardiogram with Doppler and agitated saline revealed a medium to large

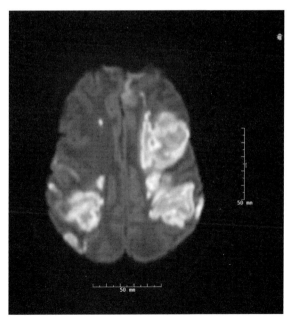

Figure 19.1 Axial diffusion-weighted MR image shows multifocal areas of restricted diffusion involving bilateral middle cerebral artery territories

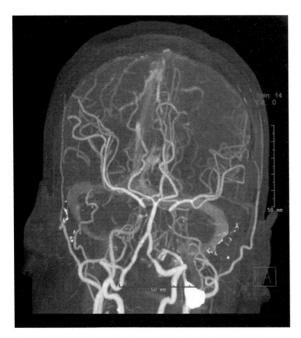

Figure 19.2 CT Angiography head and neck shows complete occlusion of the proximal left internal carotid artery (ICA) and severe narrowing along the right ICA with distal reconstitution of distal bilateral ICAs from retrograde flow via posterior communicating arteries. Bilateral middle and anterior cerebral arteries are patent. There is moderate stenosis of the V4 segment of the left vertebral artery from atherosclerotic disease.

inter-atrial septal defect with a septal aneurysm; results were confirmed on cardiac CT. A transesophageal echocardiogram could not be performed due to loose teeth. The remainder of her stroke workup was unremarkable, including an electrocardiogram, hypercoagulable panel, antiphospholipid antibodies, antineutrophil cytoplasmic autoantibody (ANCA) panel, myeloperoxidase and proteinase-3 autoantibodies, and bilateral lower extremity ultrasound. An electroencephalogram (EEG) showed moderate diffuse encephalopathy with regional slowing over the left frontal region, correlating with a stroke lesion; no seizures or epileptiform discharges were appreciated.

The rheumatology service was consulted and they concluded that a diagnosis of primary angiitis of the central nervous system (PACNS) was highly unlikely given the presence of multiple vascular risk factors and the rare incidence of PACNS. She was diagnosed with a Moyamoya-like syndrome secondary to accelerated atherosclerotic disease. With intellectual disability and dysmorphic features, it was hypothesized that RT may have a genetic condition contributing to her vasculopathy. She was treated with

antihypertensive agents, an antiplatelet agent, a high-intensity statin, and insulin.

RT's prolonged hospital course was complicated by melena, resulting in acute blood loss, anemia, and hypotension. She required transfer to the medical intensive care unit. An esophagogastroduodenoscopy showed severe esophagitis and a clean-based pre-pyloric ulcer with scattered erosions throughout the stomach. She developed additional ischemic strokes involving the bilateral basal ganglia. RT's neurological exam mildly improved throughout her admission such that she was awake and visually tracking, though she still could not follow commands. She could move her left lower extremity spontaneously; however, she was unable to overcome gravity.

Domains of Palliative Care

Ethical and Legal Aspects of Care, Social Aspects of Care

The palliative medicine service was consulted and a family meeting was held to discuss goals of care and to assist with shared decision-making. RT did not have an advance directive. RT's mother was the next of kin and she was identified as the surrogate decision maker. RT was not eligible for acute intensive rehabilitation as she was unable to follow directions as a result of her large bilateral strokes coupled with her low baseline cognitive reserve. RT's degree of overall neurological recovery was predicted to be modest at best. RT's mother was educated that the most likely outcome was that she would remain nonambulatory, incontinent, unable to eat by mouth, and fully dependent on nursing care in the long term. Furthermore, RT would be at high risk for recurrent and potentially life-threatening strokes, particularly if the underlying etiology was genetic.

Palliative Care Discussion

In this meeting, the health care teams requested that RT's mother speak about who RT was and what her life was like before the strokes. She shared that RT demonstrated a delay in developing milestones as early as six months of age; she did not ambulate until she was six years old. She was frequently sick as a child, though she always recovered more than expected. She always returned home after hospitalizations, with the exception of one time when she was discharged to a nursing facility, where she experienced extreme agitation and disorientation. Over the years, RT's family had learned that RT thrived when she was in familiar surroundings. Prior to this admission, RT was ambulating, speaking a few words, following simple commands, and performing her activities of daily living independently. She enjoyed watching TV, eating, and playing with her younger nephews. RT's mother believed she experienced joy in the smallest of pleasures, as evidenced by her smiling nature, even in the face of limited function.

RT's mother was encouraged by the small degree of recovery she had already made in the hospital, and she hoped for greater recovery than what was anticipated, just as RT had demonstrated with prior illnesses. Even if she did not recover much neurologic function, RT's mother believed RT would still enjoy an acceptable quality of life, as long as she was able to live at home, recognize her loved ones, and convey emotion. RT's mother and medical providers agreed that placement of a percutaneous endoscopic gastrostomy (PEG) tube for long-term enteral nutrition was consistent with the identified goals of returning home and making some degree of recovery. Similarly all agreed that cardiopulmonary resuscitation would not achieve these goals; her code status was changed to Do-Not-Resuscitate.

Hospital Course

After three weeks in the hospital, RT was discharged home with a PEG tube. By her three-month follow-up visit in the stroke clinic, RT was able to recognize family members, say a few words, move her left upper and lower extremities spontaneously against gravity, and carry some of her weight when transferred.

By her seven-month follow-up visit in the neuropalliative clinic, she could say a few more words, intermittently understand when others talked to her, and express basic emotions appropriately as evidenced by tears and laughter. She could also move her right upper extremity, ask for water/food, and intermittently signal when she needed to have a bowel movement. RT was encouraged to pursue a swallow evaluation and initiate intensive rehabilitation as she had recovered enough to be able to stay awake throughout the day and to follow instructions.

RT's mother was delighted with the degree of recovery thus far, and she requested anticipatory guidance regarding how much function RT could expect to regain. She was counseled that although most recovery from stroke occurs in the first three months, additional measurable improvement can occur within six months, and recovery may continue over a longer period in some patients who have significant partial return of voluntary movement.

Given RT's high risk of stroke recurrence, ongoing goals of care discussions were continued in the neuropalliative clinic. RT's mother shared that the previous several months had reinforced her belief that RT could indeed experience a joyful quality of life as long as she was able to live at home and interact with her family meaningfully. In order to ensure RT's goals would be honored, a "crisis plan" was developed with RT's mother in the event that RT suffered another large stroke. This plan outlined that RT would be taken to the hospital for evaluation and stabilization, which could include short-term intubation for airway protection due to a decreased level of consciousness. Invasive interventions such as decompressive hemicraniectomy, chest compressions, or tracheostomy would not be pursued. If it was prognosticated that RT would not be able to regain enough neurologic function to return home and recognize her family within the first three months after the stroke, then her treatment plan would be transitioned to interventions that focused on comfort rather than life prolongation.

General Remarks

Shared decision-making is a collaborative process between a patient and provider that involves integrating a patient's values and life goals with the best clinical evidence to formulate an individualized care plan. This case demonstrates several unique challenges that providers encounter when implementing shared decision-making for stroke patients. First, stroke patients are often unable to communicate their treatment preferences due to language/cognitive dysfunction and/or altered levels of consciousness. Second, the acute and unexpected nature of a stroke frequently creates a circumstance where a patient's preferences are unknown. Last, it is often difficult to predict prognosis with certainty soon after the brain injury occurs [1]. A skilled provider can mitigate these challenges by implementing fundamental palliative care skills.

The first step toward shared decision-making is to determine whether the patient has decision-making capacity. Patients must be able to comprehend the medical information presented, appreciate the various alternatives and their consequences, integrate the information to make health care choices that are congruent with their own values, and communicate these preferences [2]. A patient with the capacity for one decision may not have capacity for a more complex decision. For example, a patient may have enough capacity to select a person to make medical decisions on their behalf, but not enough capacity to weigh the risks and benefits of a conventional angiography.

If a patient lacks decision-making capacity, advance directives (when present) may provide legal evidence of a patient's previously stated wishes. Advance directives (AD) have two components: the living will and health care power of attorney (HC-POA). A living will states the patient's preferences for potential future desired treatments, including withholding or withdrawal of life-sustaining treatments. An HC-POA is someone whom the patient legally authorizes to make medical decisions on their behalf in the event that they lose decisional capacity.

In the absence of an HC-POA, the provider must identify a surrogate decision maker (SDM). Most states recognize a hierarchy of "next of kin" who may serve as a surrogate, though surrogacy order and the authority granted to surrogates vary from state to state [3]. The difference between an HC-POA and SDM is that an HC-POA is specifically chosen by the patient and is documented in a legally binding document. Surrogacy is the default process when there is no HC-POA in place, and providers turn to the surrogacy chain in a more informal way. In this case, RT did not have complex medical decision-making capacity (she likely never had complex capacity due to her baseline profound intellectual disability). RT did not have a completed HC-POA form, and therefore the medical teams identified the mother as the SDM as she was RT's next of kin.

Even when an AD exists, patient preferences will need to be interpreted by the HC-POA/SDM and provider as ADs are often ambiguous and incapable of addressing every possible nuanced situation that an incapacitated patient might be in. HC-POA/surrogates must be informed that their role is to report the patient's preferences and align decision-making based on the patient's values, rather than their own. In the absence of written documentation or prior conversations, or when the patient's preferences are not explicitly known, a patient's values can be extrapolated by exploring who the patient was before their illness, their place in their family and community,

what they enjoyed and disliked, their rationale for past health care decisions, and characteristics such as their optimism, resilience, and adaptability [4]. These valuable pieces of information can be elicited using narrative techniques (e.g., asking the surrogate to talk about the patient's life and how the illness is a part of that life story) [5]. In this case, learning about RT's pre-stroke function, experience with prior acute illness, and resilience for recovery shed light on what RT would consider an acceptable quality of life, and conversely what she would consider an intolerable health state.

Quality of life can be conceptualized as the gap between our expectations (hope, aspirations) and our experience (reality) [4, 6]. The smaller the gap, the superior we perceive our quality of life to be. This case illustrates the disability paradox, which is the phenomenon when people with serious and persistent disability report that they experience an excellent quality of life when, to most people, they seem to live an undesirable daily existence [7]. This phenomenon occurs when humans learn to accept their disability and emotionally adapt to changes in their health over time by recalibrating their internal values and expectations. Through the processes of emotional adaptation and scale recalibration, the gap between experience and expectations narrows, and quality of life is restored. Providers and patients/surrogates alike must take into account the patient's ability and willingness to accommodate, adapt, and recalibrate expectations when translating patient preferences into treatment choices.

Respecting patient autonomy has become a key element of the modern patient–doctor relationship. Providers may incorrectly interpret their role in the decision-making process as solely a vehicle for providing medical information with an obligation to remain neutral and refrain from rendering an opinion [8]. When this happens, patients and surrogates are often left with the burden of making decisions about technologies and interventions when they don't have a complete understanding of the complex medical situation or the implications of their decisions. Shared decision-making is based on exchanging knowledge, engaging in deliberation, and achieving consensus among providers and patients/surrogates. The provider's role is to make a recommendation by integrating clinical expertise, best evidence, and patient preferences. In order to achieve this, a provider must be willing to explore and acknowledge their own biases that might influence decision-making. A provider should not offer interventions that will not provide benefit or that could cause disproportionate harm. It is also the provider's responsibility to convey prognostic uncertainty honestly, while at the same time providing a helpful framework of estimates whenever possible [9]. Time-limited trials with clear clinical markers of improvement or deterioration can be considered to mitigate biases and uncertainties [10].

Once an individualized care plan has been made, evaluating outcome and assuring non-abandonment is essential to supporting the patient/surrogate in their decision. Follow-up also allows for ongoing goals-of-care discussions in case complications arise or if previously hoped health states are not achieved.

Suggested Reading

1. Cai X, Robinson J, Muehlschlegel S, White DB, Holloway RG, Sheth KN et al. Patient preferences and surrogate decision making in neuroscience intensive care units. *Neurocrit Care*. 2015;**23**(1):131–41.

2. Appelbaum PS, Grisso T. Assessing patients' capacities to consent to treatment. *N Engl J Med*. 1988;**319**:1635–8.

3. American Bar Association Commission on Law and Aging. Default Surrogate Consent Statutes. 2016. www.americanbar.org/content/dam/aba/administrative/law_aging/2014_default_surrogate_consent_statutes.authcheckdam.pdf. Accessed March 20, 2017.

4. Creutzfeldt CJ, Holloway RG. Treatment decisions after severe stroke: Uncertainty and biases. *Stroke*. 2012;**43**(12):3405–8.

5. Torke AM, Alexander GC, Lantos J. Substituted judgement: The limitations of autonomy surrogate decision making. *J Gen Intern Med* 2008;**23**(9):1514–17.

6. Calman KC. Quality of life in cancer patients – an hypothesis. *J Med Ethics*. 1984;**10**:124–7.

7. Albrecht GL, Devlieger PJ. The disability paradox: High quality of life against all odds. *Soc Sci Med*. 1999;**48**:977–88.

8. Billings JA, Krakauer EL. On patient autonomy and physician responsibility in end-of-life care. *Arch Intern Med*. 2011;**171**:849–53.

9. Holloway RG, Gramling R, Kelly AG. Estimating and communicating prognosis in advanced neurologic disease. *Neurology*. 2013;**80**:764–72.

10. Quill TE, Holloway R. Time-limited trials near the end of life. *JAMA*. 2011;**306**:1483–4.

Movement Disorders

There is a growing body of literature focused on palliative care for movement disorders, most notably Parkinson disease [1–3], but also in patients with other parkinsonian disorders, such as multiple system atrophy and progressive supranuclear palsy [4]. The protracted course of these diseases involves gradual and progressive functional decline and, in some instances, cognitive decline as well [1, 4]. Palliative care can improve the quality of life and symptom burden in these patient populations [5].

Patients with Parkinson disease experience numerous symptoms that reduce their quality of life and the severity of these symptoms is similar to that of patients with metastatic cancer and patients with amyotrophic lateral sclerosis [1, 6]. The most concerning symptoms for patients include reduced mobility, speech and communication issues, coordination difficulties, pain, fatigue, constipation, and mood disorders, leading some patients to reduce their level of participation in activities and to withdraw from social engagements [1, 7, 8].

Parkinson disease patients and caregivers have expressed a desire for improved symptom management and knowledge about the progression of disease [7, 9, 10]. The burden of caring for patients with Parkinson disease is significant and caregivers often feel unprepared for their roles and unsure about how to obtain resources for their loved ones [10–13]. Providing greater support for patients and caregivers through a palliative approach to care could ease the burden of the disease for both parties [3, 11, 13].

Given the palliative needs of Parkinson disease patients and caregivers from the time of diagnosis through the end of life, earlier incorporation of a palliative approach to care is ideal [9, 14]. These patients often have cognitive dysfunction during the course of illness [15], which may compromise their ability to discuss advance care planning late in the disease process. Understanding that patients with synucleinopathies, including Parkinson disease and

multiple system atrophy, have an increased mortality risk as compared to a matched cohort of patients [16], discussing prognosis and goals of care early in the disease course is critical.

Palliative Concepts at the Time of Diagnosis: Disease-Specific Considerations

- Parkinson disease
  - Advance directives
  - Accommodations for mobility impairment or cognitive dysfunction
  - Symptom management
  - Caregiver support
  - General considerations:
    - Discussion regarding the disease
    - Symptom management
    - Mood and coping
    - Progression of disease/disease trajectory
    - Advance care planning

Dementia

Dementia is a terminal condition and patients with advanced dementia have increased morbidity and a high six-month mortality rate [17, 18]. The burden of caregiving is also significant and it can negatively impact the health and the quality of life of dementia caregivers, as well as those for whom they care [19]. Higher caregiver burden and unmet care needs related to activities of daily living increase the likelihood of early nursing home placement and death of patients with dementia [20]. The integration of palliative care into the management plan of patients with dementia and their caregivers is an effective approach to care that can reduce patient symptoms, improve advance care planning, increase utilization of hospice services, and increase the likelihood that the location of death is concordant with patient preference [21].

A palliative approach to care focuses on optimal symptom management. Pain is a common, yet underreported and undertreated symptom in patients with dementia [18, 22–24], in part due to the difficulty with assessing pain in patients with communication and cognitive difficulties [25]. Other symptoms include dyspnea, agitation, and aspiration [18, 22, 24]. Swallowing difficulties and infections often herald the end-of-life phase in advanced dementia [18], and percutaneous enteral gastrostomy tubes are not recommended given no proven benefit of wound healing, reducing the risk of aspiration, improving functional status, or prolonging life [26–29]. Health care proxies who understood the trajectory of disease in advanced dementia are more likely to desire comfort care for their loved one at the end of life [17].

Hospice care demonstrates multiple benefits for patients with dementia, including improved pain and symptom management, less burdensome care at the end of life, and a lower likelihood of dying in the hospital [25, 30]. Family members also report greater satisfaction with the quality of care and with the dying experience when their loved ones were enrolled in hospice services [17]. Yet it remains underutilized in this patient population [31]. Early discussions regarding care preferences throughout the course of disease are important in guiding the patient's care.

Palliative Concepts at the Time of Diagnosis: Disease-Specific Considerations

- Dementia
  - Advance directives
  - Caregiver support
  - Compensatory mechanisms
  - Behavioral dyscontrol
  - Living environment
  - General considerations:
    - Discussion regarding the disease
    - Symptom management
    - Mood and coping
    - Progression of disease/disease trajectory
    - Advance care planning

Neuromuscular Diseases

Palliative care in neuromuscular disease is focused on maximizing function and adapting to the loss of mobility and independence as the disease progresses. Patients with muscular dystrophies and motor neuron diseases, of which amyotrophic lateral sclerosis (ALS) is the most common, can benefit from palliative interventions as the disease courses are progressive, incurable, and terminal [32].

Symptomatic management of respiratory dysfunction in ALS initially involves noninvasive ventilatory support, which confers a survival advantage and improves quality of life [32–34]. Discussions early in the disease course should address treatment preferences, advance care planning, and end-of-life issues, particularly if tracheostomy and mechanical ventilation are considered [11].

In amyotrophic lateral sclerosis, symptoms such as sialorrhea, spasticity, pseudobulbar affect, cramps, and pain are managed with pharmacologic and non-pharmacologic strategies [34–37]. Other common symptoms include dysphagia and weight loss, which are addressed by altering food textures and adding nutritional supplements [34, 36]. Some patients will pursue placement of a percutaneous gastrostomy tube, which can lead to weight stabilization in ALS [34, 36].

Caregivers of ALS patients report that one of the most distressing symptoms at the end of life is an inability to communicate with their loved ones [6]. Preserving communication with augmentative and alternative communication devices allows patients to remain involved in their care and it improves the quality of life for patients while reducing caregiver burden [38]. Cognitive and functional decline and behavioral dyscontrol, which may be associated with frontotemporal dementia, may also contribute to caregiver stress [39].

Palliative Concepts at the Time of Diagnosis: Disease-Specific Considerations

- Motor neuron disease
  - Advance directives
  - NIPPV/Tracheostomy/PEG
  - Accommodations for mobility impairment or cognitive dysfunction
  - Symptom management
  - Caregiver support
  - General considerations:
    - Discussion regarding the disease
    - Symptom management
    - Mood and coping
    - Progression of disease/disease trajectory
    - Advance care planning

Suggested Reading

1. Miyasaki JM, Long J, Mancini D, et al. Palliative care for advanced Parkinson disease: An interdisciplinary clinic and new scale, the ESAS-PD. *Parkinsonism & Related Disorders*. 2012;**18** Suppl. 3:S6–9.

2. Miyasaki JM. Palliative care in Parkinson's disease. *Current Neurology and Neuroscience Reports*. 2013; **13**(8):367.

3. Miyasaki JM, Kluger B. Palliative care for Parkinson's disease: Has the time come? *Current Neurology and Neuroscience Reports*. 2015;**15**(5):26.

4. Wiblin L, Lee M, Burn D. Palliative care and its emerging role in multiple system atrophy and progressive supranuclear palsy. *Parkinsonism & Related Disorders*. 2017;**34**:7–14.

5. Veronese S, Gallo G, Valle A, et al. Specialist palliative care improves the quality of life in advanced neurodegenerative disorders: NE-PAL, a pilot randomised controlled study. *BMJ Supportive & Palliative Care*. 2017;**7**(2):164–72.

6. Goy ER, Carter J, Ganzini L. Neurologic disease at the end of life: Caregiver descriptions of Parkinson disease and amyotrophic lateral sclerosis. *Journal of Palliative Medicine*. 2008;**11**(4):548–54.

7. Strupp J, Kunde A, Galushko M, Voltz R, Golla H. Severely affected by Parkinson disease: The patient's view and implications for palliative care. *The American Journal of Hospice & Palliative Care*. 2017:1049909117722006.

8. Boersma I, Jones J, Carter J, et al. Parkinson disease patients' perspectives on palliative care needs: What are they telling us? *Neurology Clinical Practice*. 2016;**6**(3):209–19.

9. Kluger BM, Fox S, Timmons S, et al. Palliative care and Parkinson's disease: Meeting summary and recommendations for clinical research. *Parkinsonism & Related Disorders*. 2017;**37**:19–26.

10. Giles S, Miyasaki J. Palliative stage Parkinson's disease: Patient and family experiences of health-care services. *Palliative Medicine*. 2009;**23**(2):120–5.

11. Hasson F, Kernohan WG, McLaughlin M, et al. An exploration into the palliative and end-of-life experiences of carers of people with Parkinson's disease. *Palliative Medicine*. 2010;**24**(7):731–6.

12. McLaughlin D, Hasson F, Kernohan WG, et al. Living and coping with Parkinson's disease: Perceptions of informal carers. *Palliative Medicine*. 2011;**25**(2): 177–82.

13. Boersma I, Jones J, Coughlan C, et al. Palliative care and Parkinson's disease: Caregiver perspectives. *Journal of Palliative Medicine*. 2017;**20**(9):930–8.

14. Richfield EW, Jones EJ, Alty JE. Palliative care for Parkinson's disease: A summary of the evidence and future directions. *Palliative Medicine*. 2013;**27**(9): 805–10.

15. Buter TC, van den Hout A, Matthews FE, Larsen JP, Brayne C, Aarsland D. Dementia and survival in Parkinson disease: A 12-year population study. *Neurology*. 2008;**70**(13):1017–22.

16. Savica R, Grossardt BR, Bower JH, et al. Survival and causes of death among people with clinically diagnosed synucleinopathies with Parkinsonism: A population-based study. *JAMA Neurology*. 2017; **74**(7):839–46.

17. Teno JMGP, Lee IC, Kuo S, Spence C, Connor S, Casarett D. Does hospice improve quality of care for persons dying from dementia? *Journal of the American Geriatric Society*. 2011;**59**(8):1531–6.

18. Mitchell SL, Teno JM, Kiely DK, et al. The clinical course of advanced dementia. *The New England Journal of Medicine*. 2009;**361**(16):1529–38.

19. Mohamed S, Rosenheck R, Lyketsos CG, Schneider LS. Caregiver burden in Alzheimer disease: Cross-sectional and longitudinal patient correlates. *The American Journal of Geriatric Psychiatry: Official Journal of the American Association for Geriatric Psychiatry*. 2010;**18**(10):917–27.

20. Gaugler JE, Kane RL, Kane RA, Newcomer R. Unmet care needs and key outcomes in dementia. *Journal of the American Geriatric Society*. 2005;**53**(12):2098–2105.

21. Shega JW, Levin A, Hougham GW, et al. Palliative Excellence in Alzheimer Care Efforts (PEACE): A program description. *Journal of Palliative Medicine*. 2003;**6**(2):315–20.

22. Sampson EL, Candy B, Davis S, et al. Living and dying with advanced dementia: A prospective cohort study of symptoms, service use and care at the end of life. *Palliative Medicine*. 2017:269216317726443.

23. Hanson E, Hellstrom A, Sandvide A, et al. The extended palliative phase of dementia – An integrative literature review. *Dementia (London, England)*. 2016.

24. Hendriks SA, Smalbrugge M, Hertogh CM, van der Steen JT. Dying with dementia: Symptoms, treatment, and quality of life in the last week of life. *Journal of Pain and Symptom Management*. 2014;**47**(4): 710–20.

25. Monroe TB, Carter MA, Feldt KS, Dietrich MS, Cowan RL. Pain and hospice care in nursing home residents with dementia and terminal cancer. *Geriatrics & Gerontology International*. 2013;**13**(4): 1018–25.

26. Finucane TE, Christmas C, Travis K. Tube feeding in patients with advanced dementia: A review of the evidence. *JAMA*. 1999;**282**(14):1365–70.

27. McCann R. Lack of evidence about tube feeding – Food for thought. *JAMA*. 1999;**282**(14):1380–1.

28. Mitchell SL, Mor V, Gozalo PL, Servadio JL, Teno JM. Tube feeding in US nursing home residents with advanced dementia, 2000–2014. *JAMA*. 2016;**316**(7): 769–70.

29. Teno JM, Gozalo PL, Mitchell SL, et al. Does feeding tube insertion and its timing improve survival? *Journal of the American Geriatric Society*. 2012;**60**(10): 1918–21.

30. Miller SC, Lima JC, Mitchell SL. Influence of hospice on nursing home residents with advanced dementia who received Medicare-skilled nursing facility care near the end of life. ? *Journal of the American Geriatric Society*. 2012;**60**(11):2035–41.

31. Kiely DK, Givens JL, Shaffer ML, Teno JM, Mitchell SL. Hospice use and outcomes in nursing home residents with advanced dementia. *Journal of the American Geriatric Society*. 2010;**58**(12):2284–91.

32. de Visser M, Oliver DJ. Palliative care in neuromuscular diseases. *Current Opinion in Neurology*. 2017.

33. Bourke SC, Tomlinson M, Williams TL, Bullock RE, Shaw PJ, Gibson GJ. Effects of non-invasive ventilation on survival and quality of life in patients with amyotrophic lateral sclerosis: A randomised controlled trial. *The Lancet Neurology*. 2006;**5**(2):140–7.

34. Miller RG, Jackson CE, Kasarskis EJ, et al. Practice parameter update: The care of the patient with amyotrophic lateral sclerosis: Drug, nutritional, and respiratory therapies (an evidence-based review): report of the Quality Standards Subcommittee of the American Academy of Neurology. *Neurology*. 2009;**73**(15): 1218–26.

35. Hobson EV, McDermott CJ. Supportive and symptomatic management of amyotrophic lateral sclerosis. *Nature Reviews Neurology*. 2016;**12**(9): 526–38.

36. Elman LB, Houghton DJ, Wu GF, Hurtig HI, Markowitz CE, McCluskey L. Palliative care in amyotrophic lateral sclerosis, Parkinson's disease, and multiple sclerosis. *Journal of Palliative Medicine*. 2007;**10**(2):433–57.

37. Karam CY, Paganoni S, Joyce N, Carter GT, Bedlack R. Palliative care issues in amyotrophic lateral sclerosis: An evidenced-based review. *The American Journal of Hospice & Palliative Care*. 2016;**33**(1): 84–92.

38. Hwang CS, Weng HH, Wang LF, Tsai CH, Chang HT. An eye-tracking assistive device improves the quality of life for ALS patients and reduces the caregivers' burden. *Journal of Motor Behavior*. 2014; **46**(4):233–8.

39. de Wit J, Bakker LA, van Groenestijn AC, et al. Caregiver burden in amyotrophic lateral sclerosis: A systematic review. *Palliative Medicine*. 2017:269216317709965.

Making a Diagnosis with Compassion in Parkinson's Disease

Benzi M. Kluger

Clinical History

A 42-year-old right-handed woman presents to our outpatient neurology clinic for a second opinion of a possible diagnosis of Parkinson's disease (PD). Her symptoms began two years ago with a slight tremor noted in the fingers of her left hand at rest. She was initially diagnosed by her primary care doctor as having essential tremor and started on propranolol, which she thinks may have been helpful. Over the past year she has noted increased stiffness on her left leg, curling of her left toes, and slowness with fine motor movements, including typing and some aspects of dressing. These symptoms have been increasing over the past six months and she has recently noted some symptoms in her right leg as well. She has not had any falls but does report worsening of her balance, slow gait, and a tendency to drag her left leg. Other symptoms noted over this time period include vivid dreams, brief visual hallucinations, fatigue, and increased urinary urgency.

She has seen two neurologists over the past three months for these symptoms. The first diagnosed her with either primary lateral sclerosis or stiff person syndrome. The second told her she had probable PD and prescribed her rasagiline, which she tried for a couple of weeks and stopped with no noted benefit.

At the time of our consultation she was married, had two daughters aged 9 and 14, and was working full time in an office job involving significant writing responsibilities. She had a family history of PD in a grandfather who developed it in his eighties and who died in a nursing home wheelchair bound and with dementia.

Examination

She appeared anxious and tearful at times during the history and examination. She scored 27 out of 30 on the Montreal Cognitive Assessment. She had mild hypophonia and decreased blink rate. She had good strength and range of motion. There was a very mild left hand tremor noted with distraction as well as a bilateral action tremor, worse on her left. She had rigidity with cogwheeling, which was worse on her left side and noted in both arms and legs. She also had bradykinesia with decrements of fine motor movements in a similar pattern. She was able to stand with arms folded, albeit slowly, and had a stable gait with diminished arm swing left more than right and mild shuffling, and she took two steps to turn. Her pull test was negative.

Palliative Domain of Care

Psychological Aspects of Care – Providing a diagnosis with compassion

The time of diagnosis can be a very traumatic event for persons living with PD and their families [1]. In fact, there is evidence in both PD and other chronic conditions that the time of diagnosis is frequently a time of increased palliative care needs and one that is frequently not handled in an optimal manner by clinicians from patients' and families' perspective [2].

Many neurologists view PD as a relatively good diagnosis, particularly when compared to other conditions they diagnose on a regular basis such as amyotrophic lateral sclerosis, Alzheimer's disease, brain tumors, and Parkinson-plus conditions. However, most patients do not consider the words "You have Parkinson's disease" good news. While there is certainly a need to maintain hope and to stress the importance of exercise and medications in living well with PD, it is also important to listen to and validate the experience of patients and families receiving this news for the first time.

SPIKES is one acronym for how to deliver bad news that consists of: Setting up the interview; assessing the patient's Perceptions; obtaining the patient's Invitation; giving Knowledge; addressing Emotions; Strategy and summary [3]. The last of these items is perhaps the most important as many patients are in a state of shock when they first get their diagnosis and the emotional impact of the diagnosis may not have set in. They are also frequently unable to process much of the information given no matter how skillfully it is presented and a plan for a follow-up visit within the next month is often appropriate.

Palliative Care Discussion

In considering how to present the diagnosis of PD to this patient, several aspects of her history are relevant. First, this patient had received several diagnoses before coming to see a movement disorder specialist. This is not uncommon, particularly in patients with no or minimal tremor, young onset, or a relatively severe onset of motor and non-motor symptoms. When discussing her diagnosis, I thus spent extra time talking about how PD is diagnosed, why I felt this was her most likely diagnosis, and how time and her response to treatments would help secure a more accurate diagnosis.

Second, she had some experience with PD in a relative who had a poor outcome. We thus discussed the variability in symptoms and progression across patients, the advances made in treatment since her grandfather had this illness, and the fact that her age made a rapid progression to dementia less likely. We did not delve deeper into prognosis as I felt she already had a lot of information to process and this was our first meeting.

Third, she had tried one medication with minimal results. When starting new medications it is important to inform patients of side effects, as well as the nature and timing of expected benefits, which are typically mild in the case of rasagiline and can take four to six weeks to accrue. Given the severity of her symptoms and that they were impacting her function and work, we decided to start levodopa to gain more rapid control of her symptoms, secure her diagnosis, and establish a therapeutic relationship.

Last, as a young woman who was working and had children, this diagnosis was both very unexpected and potentially severely disruptive to her life plans. In talking to her at this first meeting, it was obvious that she was experiencing anticipatory grief and worry for her future. These are both normal psychological reactions to the news she received and important to distinguish from depression and anxiety disorders, which are also common in this population. Both grief and worry can be disabling, but they should be tied to specific issues, unlike depression and anxiety,

which are often described as free-floating. Grief and worry tend to respond better to behavioral interventions, including validation, whereas depression and anxiety respond best to a combination of medications and structured therapy [4].

Given how much she had to process and how many issues we still had to work on, we set up a meeting with our outpatient neurology palliative care team for one month later to give her a chance to process this information, to see how she did with her initial treatment, and to delve more deeply into the social, psychological, and spiritual aspects of how this diagnosis was affecting her.

PD Disease Course

She demonstrated a good response to levodopa at a relatively low dose and found her improvement in motor symptoms very encouraging. Our social worker addressed questions she had regarding work, disability, and planning for the future, including caring for her children. She also discussed the availability of several PD-related exercise classes and a young-onset support group. Our chaplain discussed several of the difficult emotions associated with this diagnosis, particularly grief, anger, and concern for her future.

Over the next year, she became more comfortable with her diagnosis and she made an excellent adjustment. She told her boss and coworkers about the diagnosis and she was able to make arrangements for working part-time and doing more work from home. She also became very active in her young-onset support group and in a dance company for PD.

General Remarks

This case demonstrates several important palliative care concepts. First, the time of diagnosis represents a potential crisis point for patients and families. Delivering bad news, including a diagnosis such as PD, is an essential skill for almost all doctors and is considered a core aspect of the primary palliative care skills and approaches all doctors should have [5]. Careful listening and close follow-up are key components for providing a diagnosis in a compassionate manner.

Second, patients may have emotional reactions associated with a new diagnosis or ongoing changes in their health that are normal psychological reactions, including grief, anger, frustration, guilt, and worry. It is important to provide validation for these emotions and not to pathologize these reactions as psychiatric diagnoses. As these emotions may have a significant impact on patients' and caregivers' quality of life and function, it is important to address them and to work with a counselor or chaplain as needed. As psychiatric disorders are also quite common in PD and other neurologic diagnoses, it is also important to take a careful history to determine whether these issues are also present and contributing to emotional distress.

Third, there is significant variability across PD patients in terms of presenting symptoms, severity, and progression. This can make both diagnosis and prognosis challenging. It can also be reassuring for patients to know that they are not fated to have a similar progression to relatives or friends in their life. When patients have severe motor or non-motor symptoms early in the disease course, I think it is important to treat these aggressively to restore function, quality of life, and hope as fast as possible. In my experience, I have often been surprised at how well some patients do over the long run despite having what early on appears to be very aggressive disease. The patient in this case, for example, is now 10 years into her disease course and between medications and deep brain stimulation surgery is doing very well, and she remains quite active and functional. I thus typically reserve any conversations about prognosis until after I have a chance to work with patients for several months and see how they do with treatment.

Finally, the time of diagnosis may present several social and financial challenges for patients and their families both in the present and with regard to planning for the future. This may include issues around work, childcare, housing, disability, financial planning, and relationships. Community organizations, support groups, and social workers may all be useful in helping patients and families take on these challenges and reduce worry related to financial and social uncertainties. Regarding social support, patients with young-onset or early disease often find support groups depressing as they are faced with patients with much more advanced disease. It is thus important to match patients to appropriate exercise and support groups based on their stage and symptoms.

Suggested Reading

1. Phillips LJ. Dropping the bomb: The experience of being diagnosed with Parkinson's disease. *Geriatr Nurs.* 2006;27:362–9.

2. Boersma I, Jones J, Carter J, et al. Parkinson disease patients' perspectives on palliative care needs: What are they telling us? *Neurol Clin Pract.* 2016;6:209–19.

3. Baile WF, Buckman R, Lenzi R, Glober G, Beale EA, Kudelka AP. SPIKES – A six-step protocol for delivering bad news: Application to the patient with cancer. *Oncologist.* 2000;5:302–11.

4. Jacobsen JC, Zhang B, Block SD, Maciejewski PK, Prigerson HG. Distinguishing symptoms of grief and depression in a cohort of advanced cancer patients. *Death Stud.* 2010;34:257–73.

5. Creutzfeldt CJ, Robinson MT, Holloway RG. Neurologists as primary palliative care providers: Communication and practice approaches. *Neurol Clin Pract.* 2016;6:40–8.

Caring for Patients and Families Affected by Advanced Parkinson's Disease

Benzi M. Kluger

Clinical History

A 76-year-old woman with a nine-year history of Parkinson's disease (PD) complicated by several non-motor symptoms, including dementia, was referred to our team-based outpatient neurology supportive and palliative care clinic for assistance with complex symptom management and caregiver support. While her PD began with motor symptoms that were responsive to levodopa, she has been having increasing difficulties with symptoms nonresponsive to levodopa, including fatigue, daytime somnolence, nightmares, evening agitation (sundowning), visual hallucinations, depression, anxiety, constipation, and problems with mobility. She is also requiring increased assistance for many daily activities, including dressing and meals, and she is not driving. She has not had dysphagia or weight loss.

Her 76-year-old husband is her primary caregiver and he is in good health. He is with her nearly 24 hours a day due to both safety concerns (falls) and anger/paranoia whenever he leaves her. He reports significant issues with the emotional side of being a caregiver, including grief, frustration, difficulties with handling hostility directed toward him, social isolation, and guilt. He reports that he is doing well from a physical standpoint in terms of caring for her and he denies feeling physically abused or threatened. While he is committed to caring for his wife and keeping her at home, their two daughters are concerned for his health and well-being and feel that he needs more support. The patient has a medical durable power of attorney in place (husband) but does not have advance directives or any plans in place should anything happen to the husband.

Examination

The patient was thin (5'4", 117 pounds) but weight was stable for past six months. She was alert, appropriate, and consistent with stating her desires for her care. She scored 18 out of 30 on the Montreal Cognitive Assessment. The remainder of her examination was notable for mild masked facies, hypophonia, limited range of motion in her shoulders, and rigidity and bradykinesia worse on her right side. She was unable to stand without assistance and she relied on her husband to maintain her balance with walking as she refused to use a walker.

Palliative Domain of Care

Structure and Processes of Care – Setting goals of care, prognosis, disposition, safety

This patient and her family have several palliative care issues related to her advanced PD that merit the attention of an interdisciplinary team. These issues include medical and psychiatric symptom management, advance care planning, caregiver support, home safety, dealing with difficult emotions (e.g., grief, guilt), and coordination of care across her various physicians (internist, neurologist, psychiatrist) and other disciplines (physical therapy, nursing, social work, chaplain).

Fortunately, the patient and her family were for the most part aligned in terms of their goals of care, including prioritizing comfort and quality of life over aggressive medical care and keeping the patient at home for as long as safely possible. The palliative care team worked with the patient and husband and also arranged a family/team meeting with other members of her care team, including her primary care physician and psychiatrist to discuss goals of care and to coordinate a care plan.

Advance directives were completed with input from the patient and her husband, including the Medical Orders for Scope of Treatment (MOST). The patient clearly stated that she would not want to be resuscitated, and she wanted to avoid aggressive care, including feeding tubes. The medical team worked to improve her psychiatric issues, including adding venlafaxine for anxiety and depression and quetiapine for visual hallucinations, sundowning, and nightmares. Home care was initiated, including a home safety evaluation and physical therapy. Our chaplain worked with the patient, her husband, and other family members on many of the difficult emotions that arose from this illness, including guilt and anticipatory grief. While her husband was willing to accept some outside help and support, he remained very dedicated to his wife and he was reluctant to turn over the majority of caregiving duties to others or to spend significant time apart from her.

Palliative Care Discussion

Safety issues are important to address with patients affected by neurodegenerative illness and include home safety, fall risk, and driving. For patients with dementia, wandering, financial risk (e.g., scams, excessive spending), and abuse either by or toward the patient are also important to address to prevent potentially disastrous outcomes for the patient or for other family members.

For patients with advanced neurodegenerative illnesses, it is important to discuss goals of care early as patients may lose their capacity to fully participate in these discussions due to the progressive cognitive, language, and voice impairment [1]. Studies of patient and caregiver preferences also support earlier discussions of these topics [2]. It is important to also readdress these goals periodically and following major health events as patient and family preferences can change over time.

Once safety and goals of care are established, the palliative care team can direct their focus to other medical, psychiatric, psychological, social, and spiritual issues for both the patient and their family. Because of the long-term nature of many of these illnesses and the significant cognitive and physical disability that accrues over time, it is critical to include family caregivers in these discussions. The help of a social worker in assessing caregiver and family needs and providing resources, including respite and home services, can be hugely beneficial in helping families meet their goals such as keeping a loved one at home.

In PD it is common that non-motor issues, particularly those related to dementia, mood, and behavior, and non-medication responsive motor symptoms predominate the clinical picture. Of note, up to 80 percent of persons living with PD for 20 years or longer will develop dementia, making it the leading

cause of nursing home placement and a leading cause of caregiver distress and patient disability [3].

When possible it is important to involve multiple disciplines and physicians in the care of advanced PD patients. Certain medications that are commonly used in palliative care contexts, such as haloperidol or centrally active anticholinergic agents, may be contraindicated for these patients due to the possibility of worsening motor or cognitive symptoms. While psychiatric symptoms such as anxiety and depression are important to recognize and manage, patients and families also are faced with many difficult emotions such as guilt and grief that are not psychiatric disorders but normal and expected reactions to a difficult situation. These issues are better addressed by chaplains or other counselors than psychotropic medications.

Subsequent Course

Over the next month, many symptoms were improved with medical management and the caregiver and family were feeling less stressed following goals-of-care discussions and the initiation of some home health support and unskilled homecare. However, the patient continued to progress in terms of loss of functional independence and she was beginning to lose her appetite with a five-pound weight loss.

At this point, the palliative care team held another family meeting, during which time they discussed her prognosis and the accelerated progression of her symptoms over the past three to six months. Given that her goals of care were focused on comfort and avoiding hospitalizations or other aggressive care, the current care needs of the family and her prognosis, a decision was made to initiate home hospice care. The patient was very averse to discussions of prognosis or hospice (what she called the "H" word) and would become angry and agitated when these topics were discussed. While hospice was initiated, talk of hospice and prognosis was minimized around the patient.

Over the next four months, the patient continued to show functional decline, loss of appetite, weight loss, and progression of dementia. While many of her symptoms were well controlled, her paranoia and anger toward her husband were improved with medications, but they could not be completely controlled without causing unacceptable sedation and this continued to be a source of some distress for the husband and family.

The patient continued with hospice care for the duration of her illness and she died peacefully at home surrounded by her family.

General Remarks

PD patients are less likely to die at home or to receive hospice care than age-matched adults [4]. Reasons for the low utilization of hospice may include the high variability of disease progression among patients and the lack of training in palliative care among neurologists or other physicians who care for PD patients. Although there are not specific hospice guidelines for PD, guidelines do exist for dementia, adult failure to thrive, and general neurologic disorders that can be applied to PD [5]. Important signs that hospice may be appropriate include weight loss, decreasing benefit of medications, accelerating decline of function, and recurrent hospitalizations for falls or aspiration [6]. While less studied, we find that a similar approach works well with other parkinsonian disorders, including multiple system atrophy, progressive supranuclear palsy, dementia with Lewy bodies, and vascular dementia. In fact, these disorders typically have a worse prognosis and respond less well to dopaminergic therapies, making palliative care approaches even more essential in patient and caregiver support.

Although prognosis is the most visible criteria for hospice and one that determines payment for hospice services in many systems, including US Medicare, it is not the most important from a patient and care perspective. When I discuss hospice with patients, I find that it is more helpful to frame hospice in terms of the goals of care of the patient and family and the services that hospice can provide. If the goals of the family and services of hospice align, I let patients and families know whether I believe they would meet the criteria for hospice, which include estimates of prognosis and documentation of functional decline.

Discussions around prognosis and end-of-life care can be difficult and it is important to be as honest as possible with patients and families while acknowledging one's own limitations in predicting the future as well as getting a clear understanding of how much the patient and family want to and are ready to hear. In this particular case, the patient became agitated when these topics were discussed and the palliative care team worked to balance the patient and family's needs while respecting the patient's discomfort with these topics. It is not uncommon that we encounter scenarios where patients are comfortable with these topics and initiating end-of-life care and it is the caregivers or other family members who need extra support or conversations before care plans can be initiated.

Suggested Reading

1. Snineh MA, Camicioli R, Miyasaki JM. Decisional capacity for advanced care directives in Parkinson's disease with cognitive complaints. *Parkinsonism Relat Disord*. In press.

2. Tuck KK, Brod L, Nutt J, Fromme EK. Preferences of patients with Parkinson's disease for communication about advanced care planning. *Am J Hosp Palliat Care*. 2015;**32**:68–77.

3. Hely MA, Reid WG, Adena MA, Halliday GM, Morris JG. The Sydney multicenter study of Parkinson's disease: The inevitability of dementia at 20 years. *Mov Disord*. 2008;**23**:837–44.

4. Miyasaki JM, Kluger B. Palliative care for Parkinson's disease: Has the time come? *Current Neurology and Neuroscience Reports*. 2015;**15**:26.

5. Boersma I, Miyasaki J, Kutner J, Kluger B. Palliative care and neurology: Time for a paradigm shift. *Neurology*. 2014;**83**:561–7.

6. Goy ER, Bohlig A, Carter J, Ganzini L. Identifying predictors of hospice eligibility in patients with Parkinson disease. *Am J Hosp Palliat Care*. 2015;**32**:29–33.

Cognitive Decline in Parkinson Disease

Janis M. Miyasaki

Introduction

Palliative care for Parkinson disease (PD) includes care for Lewy body dementia, multiple system atrophy, progressive supranuclear palsy, corticobasal syndrome, and any patient seen in a movement disorders program. These patients have progressive, neurodegenerative illnesses that involve motor and non-motor symptoms, resulting in complex management, challenges in late stages, and a high degree of symptom burden. Traditional approaches to palliative care do not work in movement disorders patients and indeed may result in harm for these patients. Therefore, being attuned to their symptoms and management is key for a palliative care physician or other clinician who is involved in their care.

Clinical History

Mrs. Jones is a 77-year-old woman diagnosed with Parkinson disease (PD) 21 years ago. She is a retired nurse and attends clinic with her husband. She had an excellent response to levodopa 100/25 1.5 tablets four times a day, pramipexole 1.5 mg three times a day, and amantadine 100 mg TID. Recently, she notes more anxiety and feels fatigued.

Examination

Her exam reveals very little rigidity and bradykinesia and her Unified Parkinson Disease Rating Scale (UPDRS) score is 19, which is moderate. Her Montreal Cognitive Assessment Scale (MOCA) is 18/30. Her husband does not feel that anything is wrong nor does the patient endorse a change in cognition. Her MOCA last year was 23/30.

Palliative Domain of Care

Psychological Aspects of Care – Cognitive decline and psychosis

Palliative Care Discussion

This case emphasizes that PD patients may do well for many years and decades, but by 21 years' duration of illness, cognitive issues arise [1, 2]. Assessing cognition should occur yearly to track changes until the patient develops dementia [3]. MOCA is a validated screen for dementia or major neurocognitive disorder. Recall that dementia or a major neurocognitive disorder requires impairment in one of five domains (attention, executive function, learning, memory, language, perceptual-motor, or social cognition) sufficient to impair daily function. Therefore, a supportive history is required in addition to the MOCA screen.

Mrs. Jones's MOCA score from the previous year is helpful to demonstrate the change in cognitive function. Although she and her husband do not endorse cognitive challenges, corroborative history from adult children (with the patient's permission) could be helpful. In this instance, the children confirm that Mrs. Jones is having more challenges motor-wise with poor balance and impulsivity (taking risks while walking or climbing ladders, resulting in falls), and they wonder if she is managing as well as she says. She is vague at times and sometimes cannot keep track of a conversation.

Fluctuations in thinking, which include blank staring, losing one's train of thought, and thought blocking, are signs of cognitive decline in PD [1]. Given this change in function, changing the medications to focus on levodopa alone is advisable. Levodopa is the most potent medication for PD motor symptoms with the least likelihood of causing orthostatic hypotension, delirium, confusion, psychosis, and impulse control disorders [4]. Therefore, reducing pramipexole very slowly – by 0.5 mg once a day each week (that is, pramipexole 1.5 mg in the morning, 1 mg at lunch, and 1.5 mg at dinner for one week) or reducing every two weeks is advisable to avoid dopamine agonist withdrawal syndrome [5].

With dopamine agonist withdrawal syndrome, patients report worsening motor function (without corroborating change in UPDRS), fatigue, malaise, depression, and anxiety that can last months to one year. Therefore, reducing the dopamine agonist slowly and emphasizing the goal of the reduction will help patients to improve cognition and reduce any symptoms of delirium. Some patients experience a mood-elevating effect with a dopamine agonist and therefore may need to remain on a small dose of agonist (pramipexole 0.25 mg twice a day for instance). Also keep in mind that the levodopa dose will need to increase to account for less dopamine stimulation. Pramipexole 3–4.5 mg/day is approximately equal to 300–400 mg of levodopa. Ropinirole 5 mg is equivalent to 100 mg levodopa. Rotigotine patch 3 mg is equivalent to 100 mg levodopa [6].

Over time, considering the discontinuation of amantadine may also be required. Amantadine has anticholinergic effects and although helpful for the treatment of dyskinesias, may need to be reduced or stopped in order to clear cognition. Abrupt discontinuation may result in worsening motor function or delirium even after many years of taking amantadine [7].

Clinical Course

After six months, Mrs. Jones is on a stable dose of levodopa 100/25 1.5 tablets seven times a day. She is cognitively clearer, but her family is aware of her deficits. Her husband manages her medications now. Mrs. Jones is unhappy since she is fatigued and states she does very little. Both her husband and daughter report that she continues to organize the residents of their retirement home for activities such as outings and gardening.

Upon review of her Nonmotor Symptoms Questionnaire, the family indicates she is having hallucinations. The history confirms hallucinations that are fixed and not distressing to her and delusional thoughts. She believes her husband is someone else and will happily converse with him about his family and children and then ask, "when is my husband returning?" This is distressing to her husband and family.

Physical examination does not reveal change in motor function. She does seem more vague during the interview process. At this point, the family is likely strained due to the change in Mrs. Jones's behavior. Further, they have just completed the medication

adjustment and coaxing their mother/wife to persist with the dopamine agonist discontinuation. They are likely wondering what will happen next. The delusional thinking may impact the caregiving spouse who has already coped with years if not decades of the caregiving role. If the relationship is fragile, delusional thinking may result in skilled nursing home placement. For Mrs. Jones, the delusional thoughts are reality. Imagine the disquiet or fear when a stranger is in your home and your husband is inexplicably absent. Aggressively treating delusions when possible is important for the patient's psychological well-being but also for the ongoing functioning of the family.

General Remarks

Mrs. Jones has Capgras syndrome (believing those familiar to you have been replaced with imposters). It is not clear why this particular delusion is common in PD, but changes in the occipital cortex coupled with executive dysfunction likely explain the logic behind such delusions. The approach to psychosis in PD is similar to the cognitive decline. Attempt to reduce and, if possible, discontinue any medications that might worsen cognition, use primarily levodopa to relieve motor symptoms, and ensure antidepressants are not anticholinergic. Checking blood pressure is important since orthostatic hypotension can result in cognitive fluctuations. Dysautonomia and in particular, orthostatic hypotension is common in advanced PD or Lewy body dementia. If psychotic symptoms have a sudden onset, consider checking for a urinary tract infection or occult pneumonia. TSH, vitamin B12, electrolytes, BUN, creatinine and liver function tests should also be performed.

If these tests are negative, consider adding a cognitive enhancer [8–10]. Donepezil 5–10 mg qhs and rivastigmine (1.5–6 mg bid) have evidence for use in PD dementia. Memantine has also been effective in the treatment of dementia in PD and may not worsen motor symptoms [8]. Although none has proven significantly effective in the treatment of psychosis in PD, improving cognition may resolve psychosis.

If cognitive enhancers are not effective and behavior is a concern due to safety, quetiapine may be employed [11]. Pimavanserin (40 mg daily) is a novel antipsychotic recently licensed for use specifically in PD psychosis [12]. Pimavanserin is a selective serotonin 5HT-2A inverse agonist. A placebo-controlled trial in 199 PD patients with psychosis (N = 95 active treatment) found significant improvement in positive psychotic symptoms. Ten pimavanserin subjects discontinued the study drug compared with two in the placebo group. Pimavanserin was used in PD psychosis without dementia and therefore, use in this population may not yield similar results to those in clinical trials.

Mrs. Jones has a negative metabolic workup and no evidence of infection. Further reduction of levodopa results in an unacceptable restriction in mobility. She and her family elect to try quetiapine. This does not improve her symptoms and results in sedation; clozapine is initiated with excellent results and despite the requirement for monitoring via weekly bloodwork, her family is pleased with clozapine's effects.

Suggested Reading

1. Aarsland D, Marsh L, Schrag A. Neuropsychiatric symptoms in Parkinson's disease. *Mov Disord*. 2009 Nov 15;**24**(15):2175–86.

2. Aarsland D, Kurz MW. The epidemiology of dementia associated with Parkinson's disease. *Brain Pathol*. 2010 May;**20**(3):633–9.

3. Factor SA, Bennett A, Hohler AD, Wang D, Miyasaki JM. Quality improvement in neurology: Parkinson disease update quality measurement set. *Neurology*. 2016 Jun 14;**86**(24):2278–83.

4. Miyasaki JM, Martin W, Suchowersky O, Weiner WJ, Lang AE. Practice parameter: Initiation of treatment for Parkinson's disease: An evidence-based review: Report of the Quality Standards Subcommittee of the American Academy of Neurology. *Neurology*. 2002 Jan 8;**58**(1):11–17.

5. Pondal M, Marras C, Miyasaki J, Moro E, Armstrong MJ, Strafella AP, et al. Clinical features of dopamine agonist withdrawal syndrome in a movement disorders clinic. *J Neurol Neurosurg Psychiatry*. 2013 Feb;**84**(2):130–5.

6. Tomlinson CL, Stowe R, Patel S, Rick C, Gray R, Clarke CE. Systematic review of levodopa dose equivalency reporting in Parkinson's disease. *Mov Disord*. 2010 Nov 15;**25**(15):2649–53.

7. Miyasaki JM, Grimes D, Lang AE. Acute delirium after withdrawal of amantadine in Parkinson's disease. *Neurology*. 1999 May 12;**52**(8):1720–1.

8. Svenningsson P, Westman E, Ballard C, Aarsland D. Cognitive impairment in patients with Parkinson's disease: Diagnosis, biomarkers, and treatment. *Lancet Neurol*. 2012 Aug;**11**(8):697–707.

9. Cummings J, Emre M, Aarsland D, Tekin S, Dronamraju N, Lane R. Effects of rivastigmine in Alzheimer's disease patients with and without hallucinations. *J Alzheimers Dis*. 2010;**20**(1):301–11.

10. Larsson V, Engedal K, Aarsland D, Wattmo C, Minthon L, Londos E. Quality of life and the effect of memantine in dementia with Lewy bodies and Parkinson's disease dementia. *Dement Geriatr Cogn Disord*. 2011;**32**(4):227–34.

11. Miyasaki JM, Shannon K, Voon V, Ravina B, Kleiner-Fisman G, Anderson K, et al. Practice parameter: Evaluation and treatment of depression, psychosis, and dementia in Parkinson disease (an evidence-based review): Report of the Quality Standards Subcommittee of the American Academy of Neurology. *Neurology*. 2006 Apr 11;**66**(7):996–1002.

Evolving Goals of Care as Progressive Supranuclear Palsy Progresses

Janis M. Miyasaki

Clinical History

Mr. Smith is a 62-year-old man with progressive supranuclear palsy of 10 years' duration. He did not respond to levodopa. He has had percutaneous enteral gastrostomy (PEG) feeding for several years due to severe dysphagia. In the past year, he has been hospitalized twice for more than one month both times. The last stay required an intensive care unit (ICU) admission. The patient has been mute with clinic staff for five years. Mrs. Smith states that her husband speaks with her and told her he wants to live at all costs. Mrs. Smith is on long-term disability due to stress from work. Mrs. Smith has organized in-home care for her husband three days a week. They came with great reluctance to the palliative care clinic. Mrs. Smith states that her husband has to be resuscitated and admitted to the ICU and this level of care designation will not change.

During the visit, Mrs. Smith expresses her anger at the physicians in the hospital. They had told her Mr. Smith "should not be admitted to the ICU and that his quality of life was poor." Mrs. Smith is convinced he is happy with his quality of life and wants to live "at all costs." She also states that "no one else can understand him but me, so how would they know what he wants?"

Examination

Mr. Smith is mute and does not interact by speaking, eye movements, or gestures. He is wheelchair bound, is immobile, and does not follow commands. He has a PEG tube and an indwelling catheter. His wife has a paid caregiver present at this appointment and she helps at home five days a week. Mrs. Smith is affectionate toward her husband, stroking his face and hand. She states, "He is still the handsome man I fell in love with."

Palliative Domain of Care

Structure and Processes of Care – Goals of care clarification as the disease progresses

Palliative Care Discussion

This is a challenging situation where a spouse is burned out yet feels that only she will advocate for the patient's best interests. Each spouse or family completes the Zarit Caregiver Burden Inventory in our clinic. This frequently reveals that the caregiver is not able to leave the house, feels isolated, and may feel angry and resentful toward the patient. Yet many indicate they feel they should be "doing more." The goal of ongoing care for these patients and spouses is to put supports in place so that extremes in caregiving burden do not occur. Further, the conversation about goals of care is a process that needs to be revisited as the trajectory of illness changes, if there is a hospitalization or acute deterioration, or if other health conditions arise.

In this patient's case, his wife had had the conversation about "staying alive at all costs" many years prior and Mrs. Smith could not recall when it occurred. The visit dealt with how she was managing, how connected she felt with her husband, and how challenging it must be to advocate for her husband in a complex system. At the end of two hours, Mrs. Smith admitted she wasn't clear what his wishes were and that indeed his quality of life was very diminished. Yet, despite this, she was able to recognize "the most handsome man" she ever met and value their relationship.

Acknowledging the caregiver's essential role for the patient and allowing them to express fear and the reality of their situation is important. When we, as health care providers, tell caregivers what their situation is, no matter how experienced we are, there is an element of distrust if not resentment. We only see patients for a snapshot in time, while the caregiver has been present through the duration of the illness. Further, we must acknowledge that we understand population outcomes and cannot with 100 percent certainty predict the outcomes of hypothetical situations. When we offer our knowledge as our opinion, based on research and experience, we may be better received.

Clinical Course

Mr. Smith stopped breathing two weeks after our visit and his wife allowed him to pass away in their home. A follow-up call with her confirmed that she felt it was the right time and she was confident that she provided the best possible care to him.

General Remarks

This scenario demonstrates that palliative care is the prototypic "slow medicine." Conversations around goals of care and comfort care cannot occur in minutes. Mr. Smith's situation also highlights that advance directives, physicians' orders for life-sustaining therapies, or goals-of-care designation change over time and is a discussion that should occur periodically to ensure that they reflect the patient's wishes (while able) and their best interests.

A study of decisional capacity for advance directive in PD with cognitive concerns but not dementia found that those with executive dysfunction had problems understanding, appreciating, and reasoning, yet felt able to express a choice [1]. This highlights that discussions should occur early in the course of illness and that determination for decisional capacity may require more formal testing than currently occurs. Further, conversations regarding intensity of treatment should occur in the "low risk, low emotion" ambulatory setting rather than the emergency department or a hospital ward.

Suggested Reading

1. Abu Snineh M, Camicioli R, Miyasaki JM. Decisional capacity for advanced care directives in Parkinson's disease with cognitive concerns. *Parkinsonism Relat Disord.*

Psychosis and Caregiver Strain in Parkinson Disease

Janis M. Miyasaki

Clinical History

Mr. White is a 67-year-old retired farmer who lives with his wife and son. He was diagnosed with Parkinson disease (PD) five years ago. Recently, he is less communicative in visits. His wife is strained. She was recently diagnosed with a serious medical condition. They are referred to the palliative clinic for caregiver burnout and care coordination.

Examination

Mr. White's Montreal Cognitive Assessment Scale (MOCA) score is 9/30. He is very dyskinetic, yet states his medications should be increased. He does not make eye contact, frequently loses his train of thought, and peers suspiciously at the clinic staff. His wife states that he is threatening her but she can "hold her own." Mr. White also threatened to call police to report his wife for confining him. Mrs. White told him to do it and they could take him away.

Palliative Domain of Care

Psychological Aspects of Care – Psychosis and caregiver strain

Palliative Care Discussion

This situation is a crisis. Mr. White is paranoid believing that his family is stealing from him and is threatening his wife. In fact, he was holding a lead pipe and drew back his arm to hit her. Mrs. White is less able to deal with his deterioration and her impulsiveness may be provoking more aggression rather than deescalating the situation.

Due to his severe dementia, it is not clear whether Mr. White is receiving his medications as prescribed. Trying to keep a schedule of medications can be helpful to optimize motor function while reducing the possibility that delirium is due to missed or late doses. Reducing levodopa slightly since Mr. White is no longer working may be an option. If this is insufficient to improve behavior, quetiapine or pimavanserin may help control behavior to ensure the family's and patient's safety [1, 2]. Clozapine is unlikely to be acceptable in this situation due to the requirement for blood monitoring on a weekly basis. Due to the severity of dementia, cholinesterase inhibitors may have insufficient effect.

Another option for Mr. White, if his behavior improves, is to consider adult day programs for cognitively impaired individuals. Depending on the program, they may be able to administer medications during the day, provide intellectual stimulation, and give respite to the family two or three days per week. In addition to managing medications, engaging family members in monitoring and respite for Mrs. White is appropriate.

Clinical Course

Mr. White's medications are administered by his family. They decide not to force him to take medications when he refuses, but have placed medications in his favorite foods. This has reduced his intake of levodopa and he is no longer dyskinetic. Although less agitated and aggressive, he remains psychotic and therefore quetiapine is initiated. Paranoia resolves. The family is now distressed that he is very apathetic and does not want to leave the sofa. He refuses day programs and his family does not want to force this matter.

With family support, Mrs. White acknowledged she could no longer cope with Mr. White at home and applications for a skilled nursing home were completed. The family has a sense of relief with plans in place.

General Remarks

Psychosis generally coexists with dementia. Psychosis often develops gradually over time and attention is often focused on the psychotic thoughts and actions. Resolving psychosis not uncommonly reveals apathy and the true severity of dementia. Family members often mistakenly ascribe the cognitive decline to the medication changes or new medications required to resolve psychosis. It can be helpful to inform them prior to initiating changes that apathy and cognitive decline are underling the psychosis and will be more evident once the psychosis resolves.

Suggested Reading

1. Miyasaki JM, Shannon K, Voon V, Ravina B, Kleiner-Fisman G, Anderson K, et al. Practice parameter: Evaluation and treatment of depression, psychosis, and dementia in Parkinson disease (an evidence-based review): Report of the Quality Standards Subcommittee of the American Academy of Neurology. *Neurology*. 2006 Apr 11;**66**(7):996–1002.

2. Cummings J, Isaacson S, Mills R, Williams H, Chi-Burris K, Corbett A, et al. Pimavanserin for patients with Parkinson's disease psychosis: A randomised, placebo-controlled phase 3 trial. *Lancet*. 2014 Feb 8;**383** (9916):533–40.

Constipation and Parkinson Disease

Janis M. Miyasaki

Clinical History

Mr. Black is a 72-year-old retired professor. He has advanced dementia but is independently ambulating despite 17 years of Parkinson disease (PD). His wife and business partner (who provides daytime supervision) attend the clinic appointment. Mr. and Mrs. Black have been married for five years. She is a strong advocate for her husband and does not believe he is demented. Mr. Black is severely constipated, having a bowel movement once every 21 days. He has refused a bowel routine in the past. He has little appetite and his wife is concerned about his weight loss. He is "headstrong" and has refused day programs in the past. He builds things in his garage and projects spill over into the house, causing chaos and tension. His wife continues to work, but admits to being exhausted after caring for him at night and during the weekends. His business partner minds the business and Mr. Black during the day, but he is reaching the end of his rope. He states that when Mrs. Black was entertaining, Mr. Black entered the living room, dropped his pants, and began masturbating. Mrs. Black is resigned to his "bad behavior," but the business partner feels it is outrageous.

Examination

Physical examination reveals a Montreal Cognitive Assessment Scale (MOCA) score of 16/30. His affect is angry during the interview. He does not agree with the history provided by his wife and business partner. The motor examination reveals moderate rigidity and marked bradykinesia. He can rise without difficulty and he walks independently. His balance is impaired on the pull test 2/4.

Palliative Domain of Care

Physical Aspects of Care – Symptom management

Palliative Care Discussion

Mr. Black is quite mobile despite his long duration of illness. He has several symptoms that can be addressed. Constipation is common in PD and should be aggressively managed to avoid Mr. Black's situation [1]. Mr. Black is disruptive in the home with multiple projects he does not complete. A day program may be appropriate for him.

Clinical Course

Mr. and Mrs. Black were counseled regarding the importance of a regular bowel routine. Polyethylene glycol (PEG 3350) is effective and can be used four to six times a day to increase the frequency and ease of passing bowel movements [1]. Senokot may be used to increase bowel contraction for severely constipated individuals. The Blacks also understood that his lack of appetite and weight loss were likely tied to the severe constipation. Dietary changes to increase water, fruit, and whole grains, and to reduce processed foods and meat were successful.

Mr. Black is persuaded to go to the day program. He enjoys it so much that even on days when it is cancelled, he reports to the end of the driveway to be picked up. He is given "jobs" to do at the day program and takes pride in being physically able to help out. The bowel routine is also a success and he is now having a bowel movement every five days. His appetite has improved and he has gained five pounds. Many months later, Mr. Black aspirates at dinner and develops pneumonia. He dies peacefully at home one week later with community palliative care.

General Remarks

Constipation in PD is due to dysautonomia and is an early, premotor symptom (that is, occurring even before tremor, stiffness, and slowness). Thus, in advanced stages, if constipation has not been adequately managed, patients may be severely compromised. Constipation reduces levodopa absorption and effectiveness and results in dose failures. Constipation also causes stomach bloating, nausea, and loss of appetite. In the extreme, constipation can result in bowel ischemia, requiring surgery, an ostomy bag, or death.

Suggested Reading

1. Zesiewicz TA, Sullivan KL, Arnulf I, Chaudhuri KR, Morgan JC, Gronseth GS, et al. Practice parameter: Treatment of nonmotor symptoms of Parkinson disease: Report of the Quality Standards Subcommittee of the American Academy of Neurology. *Neurology*. 2010 Mar 16;74(11): 924–31.

26

Keeping Mom Home at the End of Life

Janis M. Miyasaki

Clinical History

Mrs. Rose is a 70-year-old woman with progressive supranuclear palsy for four years. She is wheelchair bound and severely dysarthric. She can speak to her children and she recognizes their faces and voices. She does not speak at her appointments and it is not clear whether this is due to her illness or because English is not her first language. Her family assures you that she will answer simple questions with "yes" or "no" and that she can indicate her preferences for food or drink. The family is close-knit and all her children live in the same apartment building. They rotate providing care for her.

Examination

On examination, Mrs. Rose is severely rigid. Her eyes cannot move voluntarily. She seems content by her facial expression. She allows you to examine her without resisting and she smiles during the process. Examination of her skin reveals a pressure ulcer with skin breakdown.

Palliative Domain of Care

Cultural Aspects of Care – Beliefs about end-of-life care

Her daughters confide that other members of their community have told them that they must take Mrs. Rose to the hospital. If she dies at home, they will be charged with neglecting her.

Palliative Care Discussion

Cultural background is important to consider when caring for patients at the end of life. Beliefs surrounding authority, medical intervention, and religion affect patients' and families' actions. Confirming understanding and eliciting their beliefs and views can help avoid unnecessary hospitalizations or deterioration in the physician–patient relationship. In this instance, the children believed they could be put in jail for providing care for their mother at home. For the same cultural reason, they were initially reluctant to accept homecare services.

Clinical Course

Wounds are common in Parkinson disease and related disorders particularly at the end of life or in a bedbound state. The homecare wound nurse provided supplies and education to the family and the pressure ulcer resolved [1]. Additionally, physical therapy (often provided by the family as range-of-motion exercises) was recommended to reduce pressure ulcer risk.

The family appreciated the suggestions and they understood that our role was to support their goals to the best of our abilities and they were not at risk of being reported to the police.

Several months after the office visit Mrs. Rose's daughter called frantically stating that she has suddenly deteriorated. Asked to elaborate, the daughter stated, "For the past year, she would say yes or no. Now she does not speak."

Mrs. Rose's family perceived her change to be rapid (over one year). Most physicians would view loss from one word to no speech over a year to be gradual. Mrs. Rose received community palliative care and died 10 days later at home surrounded by her family. They were reassured by homecare and the neurology team that this was appropriate and they received homecare resources to care for her at home.

General Remarks

Close questioning regarding physical and cognitive decline can help to clarify the situation and help to guide decision-making and other information that the family may desire. Loss of ability to speak, changes in state of consciousness, and food refusal are often signs of imminent death (within two weeks). Thus, Mrs. Rose should receive in-home palliative care to support the family. Any medications will need to be discontinued and buccal or injectable preparations of opioids should be instituted as needed for pain or dyspnea. If patients appear to be in pain due to stiffness or rigidity, rectal levodopa can be helpful [2, 3]. Others have advocated for use of a rotigotine patch; however, this may result in nausea, vomiting, orthostatic hypotension, and agitation and therefore should be used with caution.

Suggested Reading

1. Navaid M, Melvin T, Berube J, Dotson S. Principles of wound care in hospice and palliative medicine. *Am J Hosp Palliat Care*. 2010;**27**(5):337.

2. Eisler T, Eng N, Plotkin C, Calne DB. Absorption of levodopa after rectal administration. *Neurology*. 1981;**31**(2):215–17.

3. Vogelzang JMJ, Luinstra M, Rutgers AWF. Effect of rectal levodopa administration: A case report. *Case Reports in Neurology*. 2015;7(3):209–12.

"I Miss Him Already"

Maisha T. Robinson

Clinical History

Mr. RA is a 67-year-old man with a history of coronary artery disease status post percutaneous coronary intervention and progressive supranuclear palsy (PSP) who presented to the neuropalliative care clinic for further discussion regarding symptom control, goals-of-care clarification, and end-of-life issues.

His relevant history began 11 years prior when he lost his sense of smell. Over the next two years, he had difficulty with his vision and a variety of new eyeglass prescriptions were ineffective. His work was being affected by a constellation of neurologic symptoms, including near falls, and, given concern that he would lose his job, he retired early from an overseas employer and moved back to the home that he shared with his wife. His wife noticed upon his return that he shuffled when he walked and that he was unsteady. He was diagnosed with PSP six years after the onset of his symptoms, and an MRI brain revealed atrophy of the midbrain (Figure 27.1).

Over the next five years, his wife described a progressive neurologic decline including gait instability with falls, one of which resulted in a hip fracture and left him wheelchair bound. He spent the majority of his days listening to books, as he was no longer able to read or watch television, despite the use of prisms and an eye patch for diplopia. He choked when he ate and his diet consisted of soft, pureed, or finely chopped foods. He ate very little, around 800 calories a day, and he had lost approximately 75 pounds over the course of four years. Their bathroom had been modified to include grab bars, he slept in a hospital bed, and he used a urinal for convenience. He spoke very little. At the time of the consultation, he was taking carbidopa/levodopa 25/100 mg three tablets, four times a day.

Examination

He was afebrile with normal vital signs. In the office, he was sitting in a wheelchair and he appeared well groomed in a long-sleeve shirt, fleece, jeans, and tennis shoes. He was frail but in no apparent distress. There was paranasal seborrhea and apraxia of eyelid opening. His pupils were equal, round, and reactive to light; conjunctiva were normal. Marked ophthalmoparesis was noted with restricted gaze in all directions and horizontal diplopia upon removal of the eye patch. He was bradykinetic and hypomimetic. He had a severe mixed hypokinetic and spastic dysarthria, with some words being unintelligible.

Palliative Domains of Care

Structure and Processes of Care – Discussing prognosis and the trajectory of disease

Social Aspects of Care – Caregiver support

End-of-Life Issues – Hospice care

Palliative Care Discussion

It was clear from the history and the examination that Mr. RA had advanced PSP with progressive

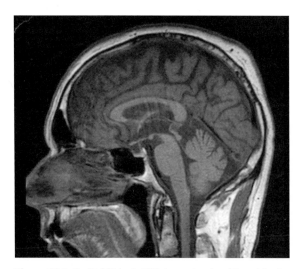

Figure 27.1 Sagittal T1 brain MRI shows atrophy of the midbrain, the "hummingbird" sign

worsening of symptoms over the past several years. He was now incapable of caring for himself and his wife and a hired caregiver managed his activities of daily living, including bathing, dressing, feeding, toileting, and transfers. He required total assistance and 24-hour supervision.

From a symptom standpoint, he was continent of urine and stool, his constipation was managed with polyethylene glycol, and he received botulinum toxin for sialorrhea. Clonazepam had been started for insomnia and anxiety at night after he began getting up in the middle of the night and "trying to get ready for work." While he endorsed a low mood, which he felt was natural given his situation, he was not suicidal. Lubricating eye drops were recommended multiple times a day and an eye patch was used for diplopia in the setting of convergence insufficiency.

During the visit, he expressed concern about the continued progression of the disease and he was most worried that he would choke to death. He understood that his condition was expected to worsen over time and he was disinterested in pursuing artificial nutrition through a percutaneous gastrostomy tube. His quality of life was poor and he explained that he did not wish to prolong it in that state, which was consistent with his wishes in his advance directive. His wife was hoping to continue to care for him at home, but it was evident that the strain of caregiving was taking a toll on her.

Throughout the course of their 40-year marriage, they had lived apart the majority of that time due to his work obligations. Since his retirement, they had spent more time together than they had spent during the entirety of their marriage. This was a significant adjustment for them both, but particularly for his wife. She was used to being very independent and now she was rarely able to leave the house as he could not be left alone. She was witnessing his decline and, understandably, that was a difficult reality for her. She was grieving the loss of the man that she married.

Hospice care was discussed, including the guidelines for hospice enrollment, the philosophy of care, the team composition, and the services that they provide.

Clinical Course

Mr. RA and his wife requested some time to think about their options regarding hospice care. They returned home and his wife called the office four days later to state that he wanted to pursue hospice. Since the visit, he had seemed more introverted and he was eating less and expressing more concern about choking. He was grieving the approaching loss of his life, his loss of independence, and his loss of enjoyment of the activities that he loved. His wife too expressed a sense of loss of the conversation with her husband, of her independence, and of her husband. She stated, "I miss him already." He enrolled in hospice care two days later and he died peacefully at home 10 days after enrollment.

General Remarks

Mr. RA and his wife both experienced profound losses throughout the course of his illness, particularly over the last few years when he became more dependent on his wife. This was a significant reversal of the roles in their marriage and the adjustment was challenging for both of them. The entire management plan for patients with chronic, progressive, and incurable neurologic disorders is palliative focused. Controlling symptoms and optimizing function, supporting caregivers, and providing anticipatory guidance are all essential in helping patients and their families cope with these challenging diseases.

He had a slow but steady decline in function over years, which is often the trajectory to death and disability in patients with neurodegenerative disease such as PSP [1]. At the time of the consultation, he had multiple signs and symptoms that were suggestive of advanced PSP, such as dysphagia, weight loss, and frailty [2]. While they both realized that he was declining, his wife was visibly surprised – but ultimately thankful – that hospice was being discussed.

The conversation was therapeutic for both of them as he was able to express his desire to not prolong his life and an out-of-hospital Do-Not-Resuscitate form was signed, which his wife thought was consistent with his wishes independent of his low mood. Additionally, his wife had the opportunity to express her feelings and to have them validated. *Forewarning, preparedness for death, pre-loss grief,* or *anticipatory grief* are terms used to characterize feelings of loss by a caregiver that occur prior to a loved one's death [3]. It is important to ask about and to acknowledge anticipatory grief as it may be a risk factor for post-loss depression or adverse bereavement outcomes [3]. Caregiver strain should be addressed throughout the course of illness. In the parkinsonian disease patient population, low mood, cognitive decline, and severity of illness can be associated with increased caregiver burden [2].

In this situation with Mr. RA, hospice care would offer myriad benefits to both him and his wife. The team was able to assess his symptoms, to alleviate his fears about choking, and to reassure him that the dying process would be comfortable. His wife would also receive much-needed assistance with his care and anticipatory guidance regarding the dying process. Spiritual support was also available to both of them to assist them in navigating the end of his life and bereavement services were available to his wife for up to 13 months following his death.

Suggested Reading

1. Holloway RG, Gramling R, Kelly AG. Estimating and communicating prognosis in advanced neurologic disease. *Neurology*. 2013 Feb 19;**80**(8):764–72.

2. Wiblin L, Lee M, Burn D. Palliative care and its emerging role in multiple system atrophy and progressive supranuclear palsy. *Parkinsonism Relat Disord*. 2017 Jan;**34**:7–14. Epub 2016 Oct 19.

3. Nielsen MK, Neergaard MA, Jensen AB, Bro F, Guldin MB. Do we need to change our understanding of anticipatory grief in caregivers? A systematic review of caregiver studies during end-of-life caregiving and bereavement. *Clin Psychol Rev*. 2016 Mar;**44**:75–93. Epub 2016 Jan 8.

The Dynamic Role of Palliative Medicine throughout the Course of Neuromuscular Disease

Joel Phillips

Clinical History

Daniel, a six-year-old boy, presented to the pediatric neurologist after his pediatrician noticed that he was not meeting his motor milestones. He was accompanied by his father, who said, "He's not like the other kids. After running and playing, he starts crying and says his legs hurt."

Examination

His physical exam demonstrates hypertrophy of his lower limbs and tongue. Creatinine kinase is above normal. A muscle biopsy confirms the diagnosis of limb girdle muscular dystrophy 2I (LGMD2I). He is referred to a local interdisciplinary clinic that treats patients with neuromuscular diseases. There, he receives care from a team of experts offering supportive care in regard to physical and occupational therapy, in addition to medical social work and other ancillary services. He and his family are also introduced to a pediatric palliative medicine physician.

During their initial visit with palliative medicine, Daniel and his family are told about his disease trajectory. They are informed that patients with muscular dystrophy often have periods of plateaus followed by incidents leading to functional decline, and a slow progression with expected loss of ambulation, cardiomyopathy, and respiratory compromise [1]. His goal is to maintain plateaus as long as possible, and strategies to achieve this were discussed with Daniel and his parents. On subsequent visits, noninvasive ventilation and artificial feeding were also addressed.

Palliative Domains of Care

Structure and Process of Care
Physical Aspects of Care
Care of the Imminently Dying

Palliative Care Discussion

In neuromuscular disease, interdisciplinary teams collaborate, meeting face to face, to improve patient outcomes [1]. This model of coordinating care for patients with neuromuscular disease has worked well in the pediatric population. Recently, palliative medicine has become more involved with patients with neuromuscular disorders. Palliative medicine teams have an important role ensuring that patients find meaning and value in day-to-day life by exploring patient and family goals. They provide support while patients are receiving disease-modifying treatment. Effective palliative care depends on strong communication and early involvement [2, 3]. Patients and families with neurodegenerative diseases have reported they wish they had more education at the time of diagnosis [4]. Knowing what to expect affords time to make informed decisions related to health care, based on patients' values. Therefore, the first visit is often educational. Palliative medicine can be described to the patient and family as supportive care that will be offered throughout the course of the disease. The palliative team's role is to provide aggressive symptom management, but also to offer information about the disease in order for families to make the best decisions regarding care and to ensure quality of life in spite of a debilitating illness. Palliative services may be utilized more frequently and intensively as the symptom burden and disease progress. Figure 28.1 demonstrates increased involvement of palliative care as symptom burden and disease progress.

Clinical Course

Over the next several years, Daniel showed a slow progression of muscle weakness. He became wheelchair bound, and muscle spasms increased in frequency. Baclofen was changed to tizanidine with good results. Over time, he developed a dilated

Neurodegenerative Disease

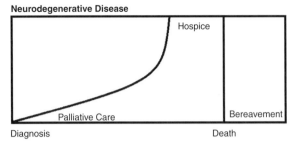

Figure 28.1 The progression of neurodegenerative disease and the role of palliative medicine. Palliative care should begin at diagnosis, providing education and support. As disease progresses with an increased symptom burden, palliative care needs increase significantly. Symptom management and advanced care planning become more important. Eventually, hospice is necessary to provide maximum support. Hospice then provides bereavement for the family after death.

cardiomyopathy. He was evaluated by a cardiologist and a pacemaker was recommended. After an exploration of goals and expectations with Daniel and his family, facilitated by the palliative care team, they agreed with device placement. A few years later, he developed dyspnea, and he required noninvasive positive pressure ventilation (NIPPV). This was initiated after again addressing goals and it was found to be consistent with providing symptomatic relief.

His dyspnea improved, but shortly after, his mother called the office. She was anxious and worried; care for Daniel was becoming overwhelming. Transfers were more difficult. Getting him ready for the day and going to various appointments was consuming much of her time, as well as his father's. Maintaining the day-to-day affairs of the household was overwhelming and they were falling behind on housework. Daniel's siblings were unable to participate in extracurricular school activities, and his parents were exhausted at the end of the day. An appointment was scheduled for the next day, where hospice care was discussed.

Caregiver burden is challenging and prevalent in families of patients with neuromuscular disease, and it correlates with the perceived health of the patient [5]. This is particularly true as parents often feel obligated to become the sole caregivers, and (due to advances in medical care) patients are living years to decades longer than previously expected [5]. Hospice is seen as the next step, for increased levels of care in palliative medicine when the prognosis is terminal. It provides support and a safety net for the family.

In the pediatric population, hospice can be offered as "concurrent care" through age 20; patients do not need to relinquish curative therapy, as in the adult population [6]. Patients can continue regular visits with their neurologist and other providers. Hospice can provide additional resources to the patients and family. Nurses and aides are able to visit on a regular basis to help manage symptoms and assist with activities of daily living. Volunteers can help with light housework, and a social worker provides supportive resources. Chaplains are available for psychosocial and spiritual support. Hospice also provides respite care, offering inpatient care for patients up to five days at a time [7]. This allows families to step away from the role of caregiver and their day-to-day responsibilities in order to focus more time on developing relationships or practice self-care.

Daniel's family chose to enroll with hospice, and, after several weeks, they reported that his care had significantly improved. His mother noticed her stress had diminished, and there was more time to spend with Daniel's siblings. He was satisfied with his quality of life into young adulthood. He was visited by the palliative medicine team on a regular basis.

One evening, he developed severe tachypnea with an increased sensation of air hunger. Settings were increased on his NIPPV without success. As per previous discussions with his neurologist and palliative care physician, he declined intubation or tracheostomy for respiratory failure. Family was with him and he reported that he was "tired of all this." Medications were titrated to achieve comfort, and he died several hours later without pain or dyspnea. His family was supported with bereavement services by hospice for the next year.

General Remarks

Throughout the course of Daniel's disease, palliative medicine was involved and the team's role transformed and evolved with time and with his needs. Initially, they provided education and support. As the disease and symptom burden progressed, this role changed. As seen in this example, goals of care are frequently readdressed and treatment choices are made based on the patient's changing goals and values. Early on, it was acceptable to have a pacemaker, and later to use NIPPV; as the disease progressed, Daniel thought intubation or tracheostomy would cause more distress and suffering with little benefit. In later disease stages, the focus changed to more aggressive symptom management and care involving the whole family. Hospice then became a valuable resource in providing these needs. The role of palliative medicine is dynamic and it can fluctuate depending on a patient's changing needs over time.

Suggested Reading

1. Weidner NJ. Developing an interdisciplinary palliative care plan for the patient with muscular dystrophy. *Pediatr Ann.* 2005 Jul;**34**(7):546–52.

2. Carter GT, Joyce NC, Abresch AL, Smith AE, et al. Using palliative care in progressive neuromuscular disease to maximize quality of life. *Phys Med Rehabil Clin N Am.* 2012 Nov;**23**(4):903–9. doi:10.1016/j.pmr.2012.08.002. Epub 2012 Oct 17.

3. Creutzfeldt CJ, Robinson MT, Holloway RG. Neurologists as primary palliative care providers: Communication and practice approaches. *Neurol Clin Pract.* 2016 Feb;**6**(1):40–8.

4. Kluger BM, Fox S, Timmons S, Katz M, et al. Palliative care and Parkinson's disease: Meeting summary and recommendations for clinical research. *Parkinsonism Relat Disord.* 2017 Jan 11.

5. Landfeldt E, Lindgren P, Bell CF, Guglieri M, et al. Quantifying the burden of caregiving in Duchenne muscular dystrophy. *J Neurol.* 2016 May;**263**(5): 906–15. doi:10.1007/s00415-016-8080-9. Epub 2016 Mar 10.

6. Affordable Care Act, 2 U.S.C. § 2302 et seq. (2010).

7. US Department of Health and Human Services, Centers for Medicare and Medicaid Services. Medicare Hospice Benefits. CMS Product No. 02154. 2016 Feb.

Considerations for Noninvasive Ventilation in Neuromuscular Disease

Joel Phillips

Clinical History

A 64-year-old woman presents with her family to the neuro-palliative medicine clinic. She was diagnosed with amyotrophic lateral sclerosis (ALS) three years ago. She has lost the ability to ambulate and she recently started using a motorized wheelchair. Her family notes that her speech is slurred and slowed. She complains of daytime fatigue and less energy.

Examination

She is sitting in a wheelchair in no acute distress. She has a spastic dysarthria and bradyphrenia. Pulmonary function tests show a supine forced vital capacity (FVC) of 38 percent of predicted, maximum inspiratory pressure (MIP) of –46, and maximum expiratory pressure (MEP) of 56 (see Figure 29.1).

Palliative Domain of Care

Physical Aspects of Care – Dyspnea and fatigue

Palliative Care Discussion

Patients with ALS often develop respiratory compromise due to weakness of the diaphragm and other muscles of respiration [1]. Noninvasive positive pressure ventilation (NIPPV) delivers air with varying pressures using interfaces through the mouth and nose instead of through an endotracheal tube or tracheostomy. It can often meet patients' goals of alleviating dyspnea, decreasing daytime fatigue, and prolonging survival. NIPPV can be used to meet similar goals in patients with other neuromuscular diseases and spinal cord injuries as well.

Pulmonary function tests are often used to monitor respiratory function in ALS. Patients benefit from NIPPV when their supine FVC is < 50 percent of predicted, MIP < –60 cm, or with abnormal desaturations on nocturnal oximetry [2]. Continuous positive airway pressure (CPAP), although not technically ventilation, acts as a splint to maintain a patent airway with high pressure flow [3, 4]. Bi-level positive airway pressure (BPAP) is pressure-limited ventilation, allowing different pressures for inspiration and expiration, set independently from one another [3, 4]. BPAP tends to be better tolerated than CPAP, as it allows for exhalation against lower pressures. More recently, home ventilators have average volume-assured pressure support (AVAPS) settings,

DATE	O-2	PEAK FLOW	FVC (Sitting)	FEV (Sitting)	FVC (Supine)	MIP
	CO-2					MEP
2/27	98%	3.84 68%	2.08 73%	1.88 78%	2.02	– 73
	36	4.82 85%	2.20 78%	1.86 77%	71%	+69
5/19	98%	3.29 58%	1.96 69%	1.66 69%	1.72	– 70
	32	3.39 68%	1.94 69%	1.67 69%	61%	+ 70
9/20	97%	3.79 60%	1.66 53%	1.44 57%	1.19	– 46
	26	3.02 49%	1.62 52%	1.36 53%	38%	+56

Figure 29.1 Serial pulmonary function tests recorded on each visit. In particular, the FVC supine and MIP decrease significantly to the point where NIPPV is indicated.
Note: Peak flow – measured in L/sec, FVC – forced vital capacity, measured in L and percent of predicted, FEV – forced expiratory volume, measured in L and percent of predicted, MIP – maximum inspiratory pressure, measured in cmH2O, MEP – maximum expiratory pressure, measured in cmH2O.

which allow for a preset average minute volume based on a set tidal volume and backup rate [4]. Breathing cycles are patient triggered. Inspiratory and expiratory pressures vary from breath to breath in a dynamic range to meet the specific minute volume, providing for more patient comfort than other means of ventilation. Contraindications for use include facial deformities, nausea and vomiting, and decreased mental status [5]. NIPPV improves quality of life, and it prolongs survival – however, less survival benefit is seen for patients with bulbar onset ALS [2, 6]. Often, a tracheostomy can be avoided, and such procedures now have limited indications in ALS, such as excessive secretions, severe bulbar weakness, failing NIPPV, or emergent situations [6].

Clinical Course

Based on her pulmonary function tests, nocturnal pulse oximetry was ordered, and when it was completed, it showed 20 episodes of desaturation below 90 percent. NIPPV was recommended. Nocturnal use of NIPPV was compatible with the patient's goals of maintaining function and decreasing fatigue in order to spend more time with her seven-year-old granddaughter. She was started on a home ventilator with AVAPS.

The patient had difficulty tolerating her face mask at night. Respiratory therapy was able to provide nasal pillows, which the patient found more comfortable. Over the next several months, she reported better sleep and decreased fatigue. In consultation with her neurologist, she began to use her home ventilator for several hours a day. As time progressed, she found that her dyspnea was only managed with continuous use. Upon meeting with the neuro-palliativist, she and the family discussed the role of NIPPV in her treatment. She expressed a fear that ventilation would eventually prolong her life artificially. The decision was made that if she developed acute respiratory compromise or pneumonia, she would be treated symptomatically and her care team would allow natural death to occur.

General Remarks

Noninvasive ventilators can initially be difficult to tolerate, but most patients report improved comfort levels with appropriate titration [4]. Different interfaces – face masks (full or partial), nasal pillows, or mouthpieces – make treatment adaptable to patient preferences and they provide for optimum comfort. Often, respiratory therapists need to visit the patient in the home to make adjustments both to the interfaces and to the ventilator settings. In particular, it is necessary on the initiation of NIPPV and then intermittently as the disease progresses and needs change.

Importantly, when NIPPV is started, physicians should explore the reasons for its use and discuss triggers for cessation. Often, the goal of NIPPV is symptom relief, but as respiratory function declines and use becomes continuous, it becomes life-sustaining. Some patients want to continue therapy with the goal of prolonging life. Others choose to discontinue treatment. It is ethically permissible to stop any treatment that is started when it is not meeting its intended goals [7]. Having frank, honest discussions about the anticipated outcomes of therapy aid in the development of a clear treatment plan. These discussions can prevent patient and family distress over making decisions when the patient can no longer communicate his or her wishes [7]. When communication is lost, NIPPV is not meeting the set goals and it should be stopped [8]. Changing the course of treatment to purely comfort measures and allowing natural death is acceptable and it may be preferable, particularly if a patient fears becoming "locked in." Some families are distressed by making this decision. When patients direct their care by articulating their choices in advance, families feel the burden of responsibility lifted.

Suggested Reading

1. Nichols N, Van Dyke J, Nashold L, Satriotomo I, et al. Ventilatory control in ALS. *Respir Physiol Neurobiol*. 2013 Nov 1;**189**(2):429–37. doi:10.1016/j.resp.2013.05.016. Epub 2013 May 18.

2. Miller RG, Jackson CE, Kasarskis EJ, England JD, et al. Practice parameter update: The care of the patient with amyotrophic lateral sclerosis: Drug, nutritional, and respiratory therapies (an evidence based review) report of the Quality Standards Subcommittee of the American Academy of Neurology. *Neurology*. 2009 Oct 13;**73**: 1218–26.

3. Bach J, Bakshiyev R, Hon A. Noninvasive respiratory management for patients with spinal cord injury and neuromuscular disease. *Tanaffos*. 2012;**11**(1):7–11.

4. Nicolini A, Banfi P, Grecchi B, Lax A, et al. Non-invasive ventilation in the treatment of sleep-related breathing disorders: A review and update. *Rev Port Pneumol*. 2014 Nov–Dec;**20**(6):324–35. doi:10.1016/j.rppneu.2014.03.009. Epub 2014 Jun 20.

5. Yeow M, Szmuilowicz E. Practical aspects of using noninvasive positive pressure ventilation at the end of life #231. *J Palliat Med.* 2010 Sep;**13**(9):1150–1. doi:10.1089/jpm.2010.9787.

6. Heritier Barras A, Adler D, Iancu Ferfoglia R, Ricou B, et al. Is tracheostomy still an option in amyotrophic lateral sclerosis? Reflections of a multidisciplinary work group. *Swiss Med Wkly.* **201**;143:w13830. doi:10.4414/smw.2013.13830.

7. Quill C, Quill T. Palliative use of noninvasive ventilation: Navigating murky waters. *J Palliat Med.* 2014 Jun;**17**(6):657–61. doi:10.1089/jpm.2014.0010. Epub 2014 May 13.

8. Curtis JR, Cook DJ, Sinuff T, White D, et al. Noninvasive positive pressure ventilation in critical and palliative care settings: Understanding the goals of therapy. *Crit Care Med.* 2007 Mar;**35**(3): 932–9.

Optimizing Symptoms before a Compassionate Wean from the Ventilator

Jessica Besbris

Clinical History

A 60-year-old man with a history of depression, anxiety, and rapidly progressive bulbar-onset amyotrophic lateral sclerosis (ALS) was admitted to the hospital for recurrent pneumonia. His initial symptoms of dysarthria and dysphagia had developed in February, and by the time he was diagnosed with ALS in May, he had developed significant weakness in all four extremities as well. By June, he was unable to swallow most consistencies, was losing weight, was experiencing dyspnea on exertion, and he had a decline in his forced expiratory volume (FEV1) from 82 percent predicted to 40 percent predicted. At that time, he underwent percutaneous endoscopic gastrostomy (PEG) tube placement and he was started on bi-level positive airway pressure (BiPAP). By July, he was wheelchair dependent, BiPAP dependent, and nearly anarthric. In August, he presented to the emergency department with severe dyspnea and increased secretions. There was no evidence of infection or pulmonary embolus, and his respiratory distress was felt to be due to continued rapid progression of his ALS. He had originally expressed a desire to avoid being on a ventilator; however, he and his girlfriend had not expected his progression to be so rapid, and after several discussions they decided to pursue tracheostomy and mechanical ventilation, which he received the next day. Following tracheostomy, he was ventilator dependent and his girlfriend received ventilator training before discharge.

The patient remained at home on the ventilator for approximately one month, during which time he developed two pneumonias that were managed with antibiotics given through the PEG tube. At the beginning of September, he developed a third pneumonia with associated desaturations and fevers that did not respond to antibiotics at home, and he was admitted to the hospital for further management.

Examination

On admission, the patient had a low-grade fever and was saturating 88–93 percent on the ventilator. On pulmonary exam, he had rhonchi in the bilateral lower lobes. He was awake and alert, and was anarthric but able to answer questions correctly by nodding and shaking his head. He could also communicate by using his right hand to type on his phone, though very slowly and with some difficulty. He had marked atrophy throughout his extremities, and diffuse fasciculations, most notable in the left pectoral muscles and bilateral quadriceps. He had no contractures, and he had spasticity that was most notable in the bilateral upper extremities. He had severe diffuse weakness with head drop, 1/5 strength of shoulder abduction and elbow flexion/extension bilaterally, 2/5 strength throughout the left wrist and hand, 4/5 strength throughout the right wrist and hand, 3/5 strength throughout the right lower extremity, and 2/5 strength throughout the left lower extremity. His reflexes were 3+ throughout, and his toes were down-going bilaterally. Sensation was intact to light touch and pinprick throughout. Coordination and gait examinations were limited due to weakness.

Palliative Domains of Care

Physical Aspects of Care – Pain

The patient was complaining of substantial pain of the neck and bilateral shoulders. This pain had been worsening over the previous few weeks, as the weakness in his upper extremities had progressed. He had so far only tried acetaminophen with minimal relief. He and his girlfriend were also noting ongoing difficulty managing secretions, which had been previously managed with a scopolamine patch and glycopyrrolate, but which had become thicker and harder to suction.

Psychological Aspects of Care – Depression and anxiety

He had a lifelong history of depression and anxiety, and was on multiple psychiatric medications. Since his diagnosis and especially since tracheostomy placement, he had noticed a sharp increase in his symptoms, especially with respect to his anxiety. He had recently been seen by his outpatient psychiatrist, who diagnosed him with adjustment disorder superimposed on his baseline mood disorders, and he had increased his duloxetine and bupropion. The patient felt his medication increases had helped somewhat with his mood, but he continued to have severe anxiety at night that was interfering with his sleep. His psychiatrist had assessed his decision-making capacity at the time of his last visit, and he found him capable of making medical decisions.

Structure and Processes of Care – Goals of care and disposition

The patient and his girlfriend felt that his disease had progressed so rapidly that they had not had a chance to adapt to his new circumstance or to establish his goals of care prior to tracheostomy placement. They endorsed substantial anxiety related to home ventilator management. His girlfriend was managing his ventilator with intermittent help from home health aides, but they could not afford around-the-clock care, and she often went without sleep so that she could suction his secretions frequently and respond to ventilator alarms. His son lived in the area, but he worked full-time and he was unable to contribute to his in-home care. His daughter lived out of state. Consideration was being given to placement in a long-term care facility, but the patient stated that he would "rather be unplugged" than have to leave his home to move into a facility. Though his girlfriend endorsed that his desire to remain at home with her was consistent with his general approach to his care, his children were alarmed and they feared that the patient's depression was driving his consideration of discontinuing ventilator support.

Palliative Care Discussion

Because of his rapidly progressive disease and the need for urgent tracheostomy, the patient had not engaged in detailed goals-of-care discussions with his partner or with his family, and he had not defined his minimal acceptable outcome prior to becoming ventilator dependent. He was now facing a difficult decision about his ongoing care, and his loved ones were not in agreement about what they felt would be in his best interest. He was alert and he had decision-making capacity, but his inability to communicate verbally and his progressive difficulty communicating by other means threatened his ability to engage in detailed discussions about goals of care in the near future, making advance care planning a critical part of his hospitalization. Assessment and management of his physical and psychological symptoms were critical to ensuring that his decisions were not unduly influenced by these factors.

Hospital Course

The first few days of his hospitalization were focused on symptom management. He was started on antibiotics, nebulized breathing treatments (ipratropium, albuterol, and N-acetylcysteine), and chest physiotherapy. Given concerns that his anticholinergics were thickening his secretions, his glycopyrrolate frequency was reduced from four times daily to twice daily. As a result of these interventions, his fevers resolved, his saturations improved, and his secretions became thinner and easier to suction. He was started on baclofen 5 mg per PEG tube three times daily for pain related to spasticity, and occupational therapy was consulted to provide a supportive cervical collar to reduce pain due to head drop. He was also started on lidocaine/prilocaine cream three times daily, and hydrocodone 5 mg/acetaminophen 325 mg per PEG tube every four hours as needed. He was started on lorazepam 1 mg per PEG tube every six hours as needed for anxiety, and trazodone 50 mg per PEG tube at bedtime for insomnia. After four days of hospitalization, he noted improvement in his symptoms.

A family meeting was held with the patient, his girlfriend, his son, and his daughter (who participated by phone). The meeting was attended by the palliative care physician, the social worker, the primary team nurse, and the chaplain. The patient named his girlfriend as his surrogate decision maker. Slowly and with a combination of typing on his phone and answering targeted yes/no questions, the patient was able to discuss his goals of care. He shared that, although he was depressed about his medical condition, he had no suicidal ideation and he wished that he could have more good-quality time. However, he indicated that, despite improved symptom management, his minimal acceptable outcome was not being met, stating, "This is not who I am ... This is no way to live." He shared that he did not wish to transition to a long-term care facility, he did not want to prolong the end of his life on the ventilator, and he wished to stay home for the remainder of his days. He did not want to spend any more of his life in the hospital. He was hopeful to remain as comfortable as possible and to have a peaceful death in his home in the presence of his loved ones. His girlfriend and his children acknowledged his wishes, and they agreed with a plan to go home with hospice care.

General Remarks

A minority of patients with ALS choose to pursue tracheostomy and long-term mechanical ventilation. For some patients, these interventions may prolong life without impairing quality of life. For others, they may pose an unacceptable burden for patients and/or caregivers, as well as significant financial strain. As such, it is important for patients and families to be counseled in advance about the realities of long-term mechanical ventilation. Ideally, patients choosing long-term mechanical ventilation should engage in advance care planning prior to tracheostomy, with particular attention to establishing minimal acceptable outcomes and conditions under which they would no longer want to be sustained on the ventilator.

The patient was discharged home and he enrolled in home hospice care. His daughter flew in from out of town and his family gathered at his bedside. They spent several days celebrating the patient's life, looking at photos of memorable moments, playing his favorite music, and reading him the emails and letters sent by friends and family. When the patient and his family were ready, the hospice physician, nurse, chaplain, and respiratory therapist gathered at his home. He received pretreatment with opiates and benzodiazepines to prevent air hunger and anxiety, and he was weaned from the ventilator. He died peacefully several minutes later.

Suggested Reading

1. Mitsumoto H, Rabkin JG. Palliative care for patients with amyotrophic lateral sclerosis – "Prepare for the worst and hope for the best." *JAMA*. 2007; **298**(2): 207–16.

2. Kaub-Wittemer D, von Steinbuchel N, Wasner M, Laier-Groeneveld G, Borasio GD. Quality of life and psychosocial issues in ventilated patients with amyotrophic lateral sclerosis and their caregivers. *Journal of Pain and Symptom Management*. 2003; **26**(4): 890–6.

3. Ganzini L, Johnston WS, Silveira MJ. The final month of life in patients with ALS. *Neurology*. 2002; **59**(3): 428–31.

The Case of a Lost Patch

Imran Shariff

Clinical History

A 76-year-old male with a history of Alzheimer's dementia Fast 7C equivalent, failure to thrive, and a body mass index of 18 was transferred back to his nursing home from the hospital within 48 hours for a non-displaced right-sided superior pelvic rami fracture after a fall from trying to get out of bed. He was seen by the orthopedic surgical team whose recommendations were for nonsurgical medical management. The patient could not follow commands with physical and occupational therapy in the hospital and he was in severe pain. The internal medicine physician placed the patient on a fentanyl 12.5 mcg/hr patch every 72 hours as the patient had difficulty swallowing pills. Breakthrough medication was with liquid morphine 5 mg by mouth or under the tongue every four hours as needed for breakthrough pain. A dulcolax suppository was ordered every 48 hours for his bowel regimen. When the patient arrived at his original room in the facility he was comfortable when lying flat but he resisted movement due to discomfort while sitting up in bed and during care. Hospice was consulted by the facility physician due to the patient's functional decline and for pain management.

In the morning two days after hospice was consulted, the patient was in severe distress. Staff reported that he was yelling "pain" and flailing his arms the whole night. He looked angry and he had difficulty being consoled. The facility nurse had given him two doses of morphine 5 mg with relief in the previous 10 hours, but it wore off within five hours. He was tolerating a mechanical soft diet, although it was difficult to feed him due to pain. He was having bowel movements and voiding regularly. The facility staff requested to increase the patient's fentanyl patch.

Examination

Vital signs: Heart rate: 102, Respiratory Rate: 20, Blood Pressure: 104/70, Pulse Oximetry: 95 percent on room air

General: Elderly man lying in bed in distress

HEENT: No thrush, edentulous, grimacing in pain

Lungs: Clear to auscultation

Cardiovascular: Normal s1 s2, mild tachycardia

Abdomen: Bowel sounds are present, tender lower right pelvic area

Extremities: No edema, arms are striking out and legs are pulled up

Neurologic: Awake and alert, moving all extremities spontaneously

Psychiatric: Agitated, yelling

Skin: No rashes, fentanyl patch is not located

Domain of Palliative Care

Physical Aspects of Care – Pain management in patients with dementia

Pain management can be complexed in general and it can be even more challenging in demented patients who cannot verbalize a pain score. The PAINAD scale has been developed to assess patients who may not be able to use the Wong Baker faces or Thermometer scale. With multiple people involved in the care of this patient, there may be variable pain assessments that are inconsistent between staff members.

Palliative Care Discussion

In managing pain, the Pain Assessment in Advanced Dementia (PAINAD) scale is used as a pain assessment tool to measure pain in patients who are unable to verbalize a pain score. This allows the treatment team to adjust medications accordingly. It is broken down into five categories: breathing, vocalization, facial expression, body language, and consolability [1]. The total is based on a scale of 0 to 10 with 0 being no distress and 10 corresponding to severe distress.

When adjusting pain regimens, the first step is to determine if the patient is receiving the analgesic and if the analgesic is being absorbed. Research has shown that fentanyl patches are not completely absorbed in cachectic patients, although transdermal forms of medication are often used in patients with swallowing difficulty [2]. Liquid preparations are also used and they are designed to be absorbed in the sublingual and buccal areas, which yields a rapid analgesic effect, unlike fentanyl patches that take hours to be effective. Fentanyl patches should be located in all patients, particularly in patients with dementia, during the physical examination to ensure that they are in place and that they are adhering to the skin.

In this case, the fentanyl patch was not found. It may have come off during activities of daily living care or bathing, or the patient may have accidentally removed it. The location of the patch is usually documented in facility nursing charts and the date of administration is often marked on the patch. Documenting the location of the patch in the provider's notes may also facilitate finding it during the examination. If the patches are not adhering well, adhesives from the patch manufacturer can be obtained to increase the degree of adherence.

Clinical Course

In this patient's case, adhesives were administered and education regarding the proper way to document the location of the patch during each shift was performed with facility and hospice staff. A fentanyl 12.5 mcg/hr patch every 72 hours was reordered along with the adhesive and staff was encouraged to place the patches in areas that may not be accessible to the patient, such as on his back. Morphine 5 mg for pain was ordered every four hours, with three scheduled doses as the new patch was taking effect.

An additional plan was also discussed with the family in the event that the patch was removed again. At that time, the fentanyl patch would be replaced with scheduled liquid morphine 8 mg every six hours with 8 mg every two hours as needed for breakthrough pain.

General Remarks

This patient's pain crisis was attributed to nonadherence of the fentanyl patch and thus poor pain control. In anticipation of repeat events, an alternative plan for pain management was discussed and agreed upon by the family, hospice team, and facility staff. The backup plan with an increased dose of morphine was devised to adjust for some of the variability in the conversion of transdermal fentanyl to liquid morphine. The as-needed dose was also adjusted to be consistent with the scheduled dose to limit medication error. Accurately assessing pain at regular intervals in patients with dementia and ensuring that the medication regimen is effective will decrease the risk of pain crises in this patient population. Of note, if recurrent events occur with lost patches with the same caretakers, then the possibility of diversion must be explored.

Suggested Reading

1. Warden V, Hurley AC, Voicer L. Development and psychometric evaluation of the Pain Assessment in Advanced Dementia (PAINAD) scale. *J Am Med Dir Assoc.* 2003 Jan–Feb; **4**(1):9–15.

2. Heiskanen T, Mätzke S. Transdermal fentanyl in cachectic cancer patients. *Pain.* 2009 Jul;**144**(1–2): 218–22. doi: 10.1016/j.pain.2009.04.012. Epub 2009 May 12.

3. Dougherty M, Harris PS, Teno J. Hospice care in assisted living facilities versus at home: Results of a multisite cohort study. *J Am Geriatr Soc.* 2015 Jun;**63**(6):1153–7.

4. Malara A. Pain assessment in elderly with behavioral and psychological symptoms of dementia. *J Alzheimers Dis.* 2016;**50**(4):1217–25.

5. Tan EC, Jokanovic N. Prevalence of analgesic use and pain in people with and without dementia or cognitive impairment in aged care facilities: A systematic review and meta-analysis. *Curr Clin Pharmacol.* 2015; **10**(3):194–203.

6. Van Kooten J, Smalbrugge M, Prevalence of pain in nursing home residents: The role of dementia stage and dementia subtypes. *J Am Med Dir Assoc.* 2017 Feb 21.

Dementia, Delirium, and a Distended Bladder

Imran Shariff

Clinical History

An 86-year-old woman L. S. nicknamed "Betty" with a history of Parkinson's dementia, Fast score equivalent of 7A, chronic obstructive pulmonary disease (COPD), falls, and two prior hospitalizations in the previous four months due to sepsis from a urinary tract infection (UTI) returned to her assisted-living facility after a five-day hospitalization for aspiration pneumonia and a COPD exacerbation.

Four months before, the patient was using a walker to ambulate. However, with each hospitalization and subsequent skilled rehabilitation course, her cognitive and functional status worsened, in part due to a superimposed delirium. During a goals-of-care discussion between the hospitalist team and the patient's daughter, who was her health care surrogate, hospice was recommended given her recurrent hospitalizations and overall functional decline. She was enrolled in hospice care and her daughter signed a Do-Not-Resuscitate (DNR) form. She was maintained on her antibiotic regimen and a steroid course. Her foley catheter was removed prior to discharge.

Upon hospital discharge, she was dependent in all of her activities of daily living and she was moved from her room into the assisted-living facility's special care unit for dementia patients. She was transferred to her new room at the facility in the evening and she was evaluated by the on-call hospice nurse. At the time of her assessment, the patient was calm. Comfort medications were ordered, including liquid lorazepam 0.5 mg every four hours as needed for anxiety, promethazine suppositories for nausea, bisacodyl 10 mg suppositories as needed for constipation, and liquid morphine 5 mg every 1 hour as needed for pain or dyspnea. Haloperidol was not ordered as it may have exacerbated the patient's extra-pyramidal symptoms given her history of Parkinson disease.

The facility called hospice 48 hours later because the patient had increasing agitation that did not respond to three doses of lorazepam within eight hours. The patient was seen by the hospice nurse, social worker, and physician later that day. At the time of their assessment, she was noted to have intermittent periods of agitation and somnolence. The facility staff informed the hospice team that she would throw things at the staff and that she wouldn't sleep at night due to hallucinations that involved her mother yelling at her. Staff members, who were familiar with the patient before her recent hospitalization, stated that this was unusual behavior for her as she was usually friendly and appropriate. They recalled that the hallucinations of her mother were pleasant.

The nursing aides in the memory care unit noticed that she had regular bowel movements but that she had not voided in 48 hours. The facility staff was concerned that the patient may be dying and had heard of patients becoming very confused when they are at the end of life.

Examination

Pulse: 100, Respiratory Rate: 22, Blood Pressure: 170/60, Temperature: 98 degrees

She was an elderly woman who was lying in bed with incomprehensible speech and who was unable to be oriented even with her daughter at the bedside.

HEENT: Atraumatic normocephalic. Moist mucous membranes. Patent nares

Lungs: No wheezing but diminished breath sounds at the bases bilaterally

Cardiovascular: Normal s1, s2, soft systolic murmur heard at the right upper sternal border

Abdomen: Soft, distended suprapubic area that is tender to palpation

Extremities: No edema, purpura from blood draws

Skin: Warm, no rashes or wounds, no mottling, no jaundice

Musculoskeletal: No spinal or paraspinal tenderness, sarcopenia. No joint tenderness elicited at the elbows, wrists, shoulders, hips, knees, or ankles

Psychiatric: Agitated with alternating periods of yelling, and incomprehensible speech. She acknowledged her name or her nickname

Neurologic: She had a left upper extremity tremor and mild cogwheeling at the left wrist. She was tending to visual hallucinations

Palliative Domain of Care

Psychological Aspects of Care – Delirium

Delirium can be common in the elderly, particularly in the cognitively impaired population, and the hospice team has to decipher the cause. It may occur in an altered environment or lack of familiarity with surroundings. As a result, changes in locations of care may be susceptible to patients having agitation on arrival. Although the causes are often identified, the management, especially in an assisted-living or long-term care setting, may be more challenging. Delirium is stressful for the patient, family members, and the staff. In an assisted-living facility there is limited staff for the patients. Therefore memory care units may help with closer observation and needs for patients who lack independence and are prone to falls. Hospice has been shown to help provide extra support in these settings, especially if patients have symptoms that require frequent monitoring and medication adjustment. If not managed appropriately, delirium may shorten prognosis.

Due to strict Medicare and Medicaid policies on antipsychotic medication side effects causing extrapyramidal symptoms and cardiovascular events, facility directors are overly cautious about the use of typical and atypical antipsychotics for delirium.

Palliative Care Discussion

Delirium can be described as a brief, sudden change in mental status that involves a lack of attention and cognitive changes that may fluctuate. It may be assessed using a variety of tools, including the Confusion Assessment Method (CAM), the Delirium Rating Scale, the Memorial Delirium Assessment Scale, and the Delirium Symptom Interview [1]. In this case, according to the CAM questionnaire the patient had an acute change from her baseline, which fluctuated during the day. She had difficulty focusing her attention, she rambled during conversations, and she was hypervigilant at times. She exhibited mixed delirium with hypoactive and hyperactive periods.

Her delirium may have been triggered by several factors, including a change in surroundings. She was discharged from the hospital to her assisted-living facility and upon arrival, she was moved into the memory care unit there, an unfamiliar setting for her. Additionally, she was retaining urine and her suprapubic region was tender and distended. She was also on steroids for her COPD exacerbation, which can contribute to delirium, and she was receiving lorazepam, which may have a paradoxical effect in elderly, demented patients [2]. The staff was concerned that she was displaying terminal delirium, but, based on her general examination, which was inconsistent with that of a dying patient, this etiology was less likely.

Clinical Course

After reviewing the hospital and facility charts, examining the patient, and reviewing her medications, the hospice staff had a meeting with the patient's daughter, the facility director, and prior and current facility staff who were involved in Betty's care. The goals of the daughter on behalf of the patient were again reviewed and as per her daughter, she wanted to focus on comfort and the treatment of any reversible conditions. A foley catheter was placed and urinalysis and urine cultures were ordered by the hospice physician. Non-pharmacological recommendations to lessen delirium were also discussed. These included limiting nighttime interruptions, engaging her in activities for a period of time in the non-memory care unit, where her old friends and staff were located, and calling her by her preferred name, "Betty."

Her medical management involved shortening her course of steroids as her wheezing had improved, discontinuing lorazepam, and starting quetiapine 25 mg at bedtime as needed and 12.5 mg twice a day as needed for agitation as quetiapine has been studied as a safe alternative for delirium in patients with Parkinson's disease. Her antipsychotic medications would be periodically reviewed for necessary adjustments or for discontinuation of therapy.

General Remarks

The assisted-living staff depends on hospice and palliative care staff for their knowledge about patients with complex symptom needs and/or who may be near the end of life. Hospice teams advise and make recommendations to facility staff regarding treatment options and they collaborate with the patients' other care providers. Ongoing discussions between hospice and facility directors help foster a professional and educational relationship between the groups as they collectively provide care for the patients.

The management of delirium involves both pharmacologic and non-pharmacologic approaches. In this case, the placement of a foley catheter was the initial intervention as her bladder distension was most certainly a primary cause of her delirium. Quetiapine was added to her regimen given her behavioral dyscontrol as she was throwing objects and interrupting her activities of daily living, thus putting both herself and other people at potential risk of harm. The Centers for Medicare and Medicaid Services (CMS) closely monitor antipsychotics and Betty's medications were ordered for an appropriate CMS diagnosis – brief psychotic disorder. Documentation of the effect of all treatments is essential to justify the rationale for increasing, decreasing, or adding medications.

Betty improved with the interventions that were initiated. Had her delirium not responded to the treatment plan, the hospice team could have provided an escalation in the level of care in the form of hospice continuous care or Betty could have been transferred to the hospice inpatient unit if her symptoms worsened despite medical management.

Suggested Reading

1. Casarett DJ, Inouye SK. Diagnosis and management of delirium near the end of life. *Annals of Internal Medicine.* 2001;**135**(1):32–40.

2. Lonergan E, Luxenberg, J. Benzodiazepines for delirium. *Cochrane Database Systematic Review.* 2009 Oct 7.CD006379.

3. Hshieh TT, Yue J, Effectiveness of multicomponent nonpharmacological delirium interventions: A meta-analysis. *JAMA Intern Med.* 2015 Apr;**175**(4): 512–20.

4. Markowitz, J, Narasimhan, M. Delirium and antipsychotics: A systematic review of epidemiology and somatic treatment options. *Psychiatry (Edgmont).* 2008 Oct;**5**(10):29–36.

5. Ozbolt LB, Paniagua MA, Kaiser RM. Atypical antipsychotics for the treatment of delirious elders. *J Am Med Dir Assoc.* 2008 Jan;**9**(1):18–28.

6. Rao, S, Ferris, FD, Irwin, SA. Ease of screening for depression and delirium in patients enrolled in inpatient hospice care. *J Palliat Med.* 2011 Mar;**14**(3): 275–9.

7. Susan B, LeGrand, MD, Delirium in palliative medicine: A review. *Journal of Pain and Symptom Management.* 2012 Oct;**44**(4):583–94.

8. Video: Severity & scope guidance – antipsychotic medication use in nursing homes. http://surveyor training.cms.hhs.gov/pubs/VideoInformation.aspx? id=40&cid=0CMSAPSYMEDUNH_SASG.

High-grade gliomas pose significant challenges for patients and caregivers [1, 2]. At the time of diagnosis, concerns regarding function and life expectancy are prevalent and as the disease progresses, these issues become more salient. Additionally, the symptom burden tends to worsen over time, necessitating the use of pharmacological and non-pharmacological approaches to care.

The most common symptoms in patients with high-grade brain tumors are headaches, seizures, delirium, gait instability, dysphagia, focal neurological deficits, and cognitive decline [1, 3, 4]. In those who are admitted to an inpatient neurology unit, gait impairment, cognitive or personality changes, motor deficits, seizures, and delirium were the most common diagnoses [1, 5]. Caregivers also report fatigue, reduced consciousness, and aphasia as very prominent symptoms [2]. Given the communication and cognitive difficulties, along with high symptom burden, some caregivers demonstrate burnout and poor quality of life [2].

Despite the fact that malignant brain tumors are incurable, communication regarding prognosis may not be as effective as it could be, thus potentially contributing to delayed discussions and preparation for the end of life [6]. Earlier goals-of-care conversations are recommended as cognitive dysfunction later in the disease may preclude meaningful discussions [7, 8]. Inpatient hospitalizations within weeks of death are common and hospice referral in this population is often late, when patients are nonambulatory, uncommunicative, unresponsive, and within a week of death [1, 5, 9].

> **Palliative Concepts at the Time of Diagnosis: Disease-Specific Considerations**
>
> - Brain tumor
>   - Advance directives
>   - Prognostication
>   - Tumor-specific treatment options, risks/benefits/side effects
>   - Accommodations for mobility impairment or cognitive dysfunction
>   - Symptom management
>   - Caregiver support
>   - General considerations:
>   - Discussion regarding the disease
>   - Symptom management
>   - Mood and coping
>   - Progression of disease/disease trajectory
>   - Advance care planning

Suggested Reading

1. Gofton TE, Graber J, Carver A. Identifying the palliative care needs of patients living with cerebral tumors and metastases: a retrospective analysis. *Journal of Neuro-oncology.* 2012;**108**(3):527–34.

2. Flechl B, Ackerl M, Sax C, et al. The caregivers' perspective on the end-of-life phase of glioblastoma patients. *Journal of Neuro-oncology.* 2013;**112**(3):403–11.

3. Walbert T, Khan M. End-of-life symptoms and care in patients with primary malignant brain tumors: A systematic literature review. *Journal of Neuro-oncology.* 2014;**117**(2):217–24.

4. Sizoo EM, Braam L, Postma TJ, et al. Symptoms and problems in the end-of-life phase of high-grade glioma patients. *Neuro-oncology.* 2010;**12**(11):1162–6.

5. Diamond EL, Panageas KS, Dallara A, et al. Frequency and predictors of acute hospitalization before death in patients with glioblastoma. *Journal of Pain and Symptom Management.* 2017;**53**(2):257–64.

6. Diamond EL, Corner GW, De Rosa A, Breitbart W, Applebaum AJ. Prognostic awareness and communication of prognostic information in malignant glioma: A systematic review. *Journal of Neuro-oncology.* 2014;**119**(2):227–34.

7. Sizoo EM, Pasman HR, Buttolo J, et al. Decision-making in the end-of-life phase of high-grade glioma patients.

European Journal of Cancer (Oxford, England: 1990). 2012;**48**(2):226–32.

8. Sizoo EM, Taphoorn MJ, Uitdehaag B, et al. The end-of-life phase of high-grade glioma patients: Dying with dignity? *The Oncologist.* 2013;**18**(2):198–203.

9. Diamond EL, Russell D, Kryza-Lacombe M, et al. Rates and risks for late referral to hospice in patients with primary malignant brain tumors. *Neuro-oncology.* 2016;**18**(1):78–86.

"I Don't Want to Be a Burden on My Family"

Chapter

33

Kimberly Chow

Clinical History

JJ was a 49-year-old woman in her usual state of health when she began developing forgetfulness, dull bifrontal headaches, and lightheadedness. CT and MRI of the brain confirmed a 5 cm mass in the splenium of the corpus callosum with associated edema (Figure 33.1). A biopsy was performed and the pathology was consistent with primary CNS lymphoma. Further workup showed diffuse marrow uptake, but no systemic evidence of disease.

At her first neuro-oncology visit, JJ continued to report memory loss, headache, and lightheadedness. She also presented with a significant level of anxiety and depression that she related to her diagnosis. She was connected with the outpatient psychiatry service and after a long discussion with her family and oncologist, JJ confirmed her wishes to begin disease-targeted therapy. She began rituximab, methotrexate, procarbazine, and vincristine (R-MVP) with plans to follow this treatment regimen with high-dose thiotepa, busulfan, cyclophosphamide (TBC), and an autologous stem-cell transplant. After eight doses of R-MVP she was found to have a 99 percent tumor

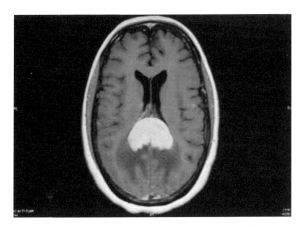

Figure 33.1 Axial T1 MRI of the brain with gadolinium shows a 5 cm mass in the splenium of the corpus callosum with associated vasogenic edema

response to treatment and her memory loss and headaches improved. significantly.

Prior to her planned admission for transplant, JJ's oncologist presented her case to the stem cell transplant case conference out of concern for JJ's emotional lability. At various clinic appointments, JJ was tearful, anxious, and expressing fear that she would be a burden on her family. At times she even stated that she did not want to proceed with transplant and would prefer to die. These complaints were assessed by psychiatry and she was deemed not at risk of harming herself or others. It was decided during the case conference that it would not be ethically appropriate to proceed with transplant if the patient felt forced. A family conference including JJ, her husband, her two children, the neuro-oncologist, the transplant physician, and the psychiatrist was held to discuss the plan of care moving forward. The risks and benefits of transplant were discussed as well as the concerns of both the oncology teams and JJ's family regarding her emotional distress. After much discussion and thought, JJ clearly stated her awareness of her behavior and that she understood a transplant was her primary chance at survival and cure of illness. She expressed fear about having to stay in the hospital for a transplant, but she felt confident that the support from her family, oncology teams, psychiatrist, and social worker would get her through the treatment.

JJ was admitted for high-dose chemotherapy and stem cell transplant the following weekend. Throughout the course of her hospitalization, she remained emotionally labile, dysphoric, and at times agitated. She also developed acute and agitated delirium secondary to steroid use, requiring a neuroleptic and benzodiazepine combination regimen. Family would take turns staying with JJ and a 1:1 companion was present to ensure safety at night if family could not stay. The Palliative Medicine Service was consulted to assist with severe pain from mucositis and chemotherapy-induced neuropathy that JJ described as intolerable suffering.

115

Examination

Alert and oriented. Able to state year and day of the week, but had difficulty with the month and exact date. Some difficulty with serial 7's. Muscle strength and tone were normal for all extremities with no evidence of atrophy. Sensation to light touch intact. Gait steady.

Palliative Domains of Care

Physical Aspects of Care

On assessment, JJ reported "8 out of 10" mouth and throat pain as well as "5 out of 10" burning pain in her hands and feet that had been present since the initial cycles of chemotherapy. Due to her inability to swallow, she was started on a low dose of morphine administered through an intravenous patient-controlled analgesic (PCA) pump, which caused sedation and little pain relief. In addition to her pain, JJ reported ongoing feelings of sadness, extreme fatigue, and worry about the future.

Psychological and Social Aspects of Care

Prior to JJ's diagnosis, she was a highly functioning middle school teacher and provider for her family, which included her husband, son, and daughter. She was born in India and immigrated to the United States with her husband in the 1980s. Per her family, JJ had no history of depression, anxiety, or paranoia. She was very involved in her religious and social community. There was no history of alcohol, drug, or tobacco use.

Ethical and Legal Aspects of Care

Her ongoing distress and agitation were upsetting for her husband, children, and care providers. Her family verbalized distress from hearing JJ cry out throughout the day and sometimes stating that she was being held against her wishes. Whenever the transplant or psychiatry team would respond to JJ's distress call, she could state the goals of treatment calmly and acknowledge her erratic behaviors.

Palliative Care Discussion

Primary CNS lymphoma is a potentially curable disease. High-dose methotrexate-based chemotherapy is currently the mainstay of treatment; however, rates of relapse are high. Increasing attention has been paid to the use of R-MPV followed by high-dose chemotherapy and autologous stem-cell transplant for this patient population with promising early outcomes [1]. Despite the curable nature of this disease, the length and intensity of treatment, which includes high-dose chemotherapy and prolonged inpatient admission following transplant, can certainly affect quality of life.

Prior to her diagnosis, JJ did not exhibit any evidence of psychiatric disorder or instability. These symptoms may have been triggered by the nature of her primary high-grade brain tumor and exacerbated by treatment. In this case, the medical oncology teams offered clear communication of risks and benefits at diagnosis and at various points of treatment. Members of the interdisciplinary team (IDT) were also incorporated into JJ's care early on in order to ensure full support and management of her psychosocial and physical needs.

Symptom clusters that include depression, anxiety, fatigue, dyspnea, and pain have been reported in patients with hematologic malignancies, including lymphoma. When these symptoms present together, they can cause a high level of distress for patients and families. A multimodal approach to care that includes both pharmacologic and non-pharmacologic approaches has been associated with improved outcomes [2]. In JJ's case, her mucositis and peripheral neuropathy were suboptimally controlled on a morphine PCA with side effects of sedation. After a full palliative care assessment and discussion with the oncology and psychiatry teams, she was rotated to a fentanyl PCA, which offered immediate relief of her pain without side effects. The psychiatry team recommended gabapentin for the treatment of both neuropathic pain and anxiety. Additional recommended interventions included providing orienting materials such as pictures of family, limited nighttime interruptions of sleep, increased daytime activity, and early mobility to target fatigue and intermittent delirium. JJ responded well to the majority of these interventions.

A recurrent theme throughout JJ's treatment was the fear of burdening her family and a desire to stop treatment rather than to continue on in emotional and physical distress. A patient's cognitive capacity to make important decisions about his/her care may be influenced by various aspects of illness, including emotional overload, fatigue, uncontrolled symptoms, medications, and overall clinical condition. Families who take on the role of surrogate decision maker should be encouraged to advocate for what they believe the patient would want for him/herself [3].

Documented discussions at various oncology visits that included JJ and her family clearly indicated her strong desire for cure and more time with her family and friends. These vital discussions allowed all family members and clinicians to feel confident that continuing on with disease-targeted therapy was ethically appropriate and consistent with JJ's goals.

Hospital Course

JJ's emotional distress continued throughout her hospitalization and it slowly improved as she recovered from her post-transplant pancytopenia. During her last inpatient week, JJ was ambulating around the hallway and interacting more with her family and staff members. She continued to verbalize feeling concerned about her overall disease and her course to recovery. These feelings were acknowledged and validated by all team members.

On the day of her discharge, JJ and her family expressed gratitude for the care provided. JJ was set up with weekly clinic visits with the transplant team and with her psychiatrist for ongoing post-transplant management and support.

General Remarks

The care for patients with primary or metastatic brain tumors must be interdisciplinary and carefully considered. Changes in personality, mood, and behavior are common and can be highly distressful for patients and their family.

A key step the oncology team took was ensuring multiple family conferences throughout the course of treatment. By clearly discussing the risks and benefits of treatments that involve high-dose chemotherapy and transplant, clinicians offer families the opportunity to hear the patients' concerns and fears as well as their values and preferences for care. This can help guide crucial treatment decisions when necessary. Additionally, the transplant team incorporated the support of various interdisciplinary team members, including psychiatry, palliative care, social work, pharmacy, and rehabilitative medicine in order to truly provide comprehensive cancer care to JJ and her family.

Suggested Reading

1. Omuro A, Correa DD, DeAngelis LM, et al. R-MPV followed by high-dose chemotherapy with TBC and autologous stem-cell transplant for newly diagnosed primary CNS lymphoma. *Blood*. 2015;**125**:1403–10.

2. Albrecht, TA. Symptom clusters in various solid tumors and hematologic malignancies. In Dahlin C, Coyne PJ, Ferrell BR, eds. *Advanced Practice Palliative Nursing*. New York: Oxford University Press, 2016, 345–56.

3. Epstein RM, Entwistle VS. Capacity and shared decision making in serious illness. In Quill TE, Miller FG, eds. *Palliative Care and Ethics*. New York: Oxford University Press, 2014, 162–86.

Palliative Amputation for Refractory Pain

34

Kimberly Chow

Clinical History

MS was a 62-year-old woman with epitheloid sarcoma of the right forearm and metastatic disease to the right axilla, lymph nodes, liver, lung, and brain. She was initially treated with multiple lines of chemotherapy and radiation therapy to the original tumor site. She was admitted to the hospital for worsening severe right shoulder and chest wall pain radiating down her entire arm and unrelieved by escalating doses of opioids.

Prior to her hospitalization, MS was followed closely in the palliative medicine clinic for pain, originally at the antecubital space from tumor involvement. She described the pain as throbbing, tingling, and with a "pins-and-needles" sensation. As her disease continued to progress and involve the right axilla and lymph nodes, she began developing severe edema from the right shoulder to her hand. Lymphedema therapy offered some feeling of support and relief. Overall, MS's pain was suboptimally controlled with a home analgesic regimen that included methadone, gabapentin, and oxycodone immediate release as needed. She required approximately six breakthrough doses per day with little relief. She denied any dose-limiting side effects

Examination

MS's neurologic exam was grossly normal with the exception of weakness and decreased sensation to touch of the entire right upper extremity (RUE). She was unable to lift her RUE against gravity and had minimal movement of all five digits.

A CT of the chest revealed increased extensive right axillary adenopathy including a 4.7 x 3.1 cm nodal mass and right supraclavicular adenopathy. She also had extensive tumor partially imaged in the RUE with diffuse edema.

An MRI of the brachial plexus showed extensive infiltrative metastases occupying the visualized musculature of the upper arm with extensive infiltration of the right axilla and chest wall. There was encasement of the brachial plexus and axillary neurovascular bundle. Rotator cuff muscles, muscles of the arm, and pectoralis musculature were also involved with tumor.

Palliative Domains of Care

Physical Aspects of Care

MS was seen for initial inpatient palliative care consultation in the urgent care center, where she was tearfully reporting severe "10 out of 10" pain to her entire RUE. She verbalized severe distress related to her pain that limited her ability to be mobile and interactive with friends and family in her life. Most of her days were spent in bed with her RUE supported by pillows in order to minimize movement and the sensation of "gravity pulling down on me." She identified sharp and burning pain that started at her right chest wall and radiated to her shoulder and fingertips in a "shooting" sensation. At best she rated her pain as "7 out of 10" after a breakthrough dose of oxycodone and with elevation. She reported occasional constipation with opioids and she denied sedation, confusion, hallucinations, or myoclonus. Her last bowel movement was the day before admission.

Psychological and Social Aspects of Care

In addition to her physical pain, MS also reported severe emotional distress from the recent death of her 32-year-old son one year prior in a motor vehicle crash. She stated how difficult it was trying to cope with both her cancer progression and the sudden loss of her son. She had another adult son who was alive and well. Both her son and her husband were extremely supportive and her husband accompanied her to all clinic and hospital visits.

Spiritual Aspects of Care

When asked about her faith and spirituality, she stated, "I'm Catholic, but it's been really hard to maintain hope recently."

Ethical and Legal Aspects of Care

MS appointed her husband as her durable power of attorney for health care.

Palliative Care Discussion

Neuropathic pain is classified as pain that arises from damage to the peripheral or central nervous system [1]. It is often underdiagnosed and undertreated, with prevalence ranging between 19 and 40 percent in various studies [2, 3]. Patients often describe this type of pain as burning, shooting, electrical, numbness, and tingling. Typical management strategies include a combination of adjuvant analgesics and opioids, although adjuvants such as antidepressants and antiepileptics are the mainstay of treatment for chronic neuropathic pain [1, 4].

In MS's case, traditional combinations of pharmacologic interventions, including gabapentin, methadone, and oxycodone, were not alleviating her pain. Given the extensive tumor burden in the RUE and chest wall and rapid progression of disease, her pain was classified as a mix of somatic and neuropathic components. Additionally, the recent death of her young son was adding to her overall distress and total pain and could not be ignored.

Hospital Course

MS had a one-month hospital course that was focused primarily on pain and symptom management. At initial consultation, her methadone dose was titrated based on breakthrough opioid use at home. She was continued on maximum doses of gabapentin and initiated on a hydromorphone intravenous patient-controlled analgesia (PCA) pump for faster relief and opioid dose-finding. The oncology team also consulted orthopedic/neurosurgery as well as the anesthesia pain service for possible interventional methods of pain relief. Social work and chaplaincy consults were placed to offer additional psychosocial and spiritual support for this patient with severe distress. A psychiatry consult was ultimately placed to assist with anxiety, depression, and complicated grief from the death of her son.

Despite rapid escalation of opioids, trials of steroids, and ketamine infusions, MS's uncontrolled pain persisted. Based on available imaging and assessment of the patient, the surgical team recommended a palliative right forequarter amputation for symptomatic relief of her severe, refractory pain. Multiple family meetings including MS, her husband, son, daughter-in-law,

palliative care, oncology, and social work helped to identify MS's goals and preferences for care. She consistently verbalized her goals of spending more time with family and having her pain controlled enough to enjoy activities outside of her house. From the oncologist's perspective, the other sites of her metastatic disease had been relatively well controlled with previous disease-targeted therapies. Options including amputation, brachial plexus nerve block, further escalation of opioids, and palliative sedation were extensively explored. With the assistance of the entire clinical team, MS decided to move forward with amputation.

Post-surgically, MS recovered remarkably well without any postoperative complications. Her pain and opioid use significantly decreased and MS described this as "a sudden relief of the pressure and weight from my arm." She began ambulating in the hallway with her husband within two days and stated that she had not walked more than one city block in nearly four months due to pain. Shortly after her surgery, MS began to report new RUE pain that she described as phantom-limb sensations; however, this pain was not nearly as severe as her previous pains and she was discharged on decreased doses of methadone and hydromorphone.

MS was followed as an outpatient by oncology, palliative care, and psychiatry. She was able to continue on disease-targeted therapies and remain active for another six months. As her disease continued to progress, MS's oncology and palliative care teams worked to smoothly transition her to home hospice care. Her phantom-limb pain was well controlled with lowered doses of methadone and therapeutic doses of gabapentin.

General Remarks

This case highlights a patient who was suffering in various domains of her life. This required an interdisciplinary team approach to care to meet MS and her family's needs throughout the course of her illness and into bereavement. Use of palliative amputation in advanced cancer is controversial depending on estimated prognosis and predicted surgical outcomes. In MS's case, this extensive surgery improved her overall quality of life and prolonged her survival. The role of palliative care specialists is to first and foremost help to identify a patient's goals, values, and preferences in the context of their life and illness. This serves as a guide in making reasonable treatment decisions that are most in line with the patient's wishes.

Suggested Reading

1. International Association for the Study of Pain (IASP). Diagnosis and classification of neuropathic pain. 2010. www.iasp-pain.org/PublicationsNews/NewsletterIssue.aspx?ItemNumber=2083. Accessed March 23, 2017.

2. Bennett MI, Rayment C, Hjermstad M, et al. Prevalence and aetiology of neuropathic pain in cancer patients: A systematic review. *Pain*. 2011;**153**:359–65.

3. Rayment C, Hjermstad MJ, Aass N, et al. Neuropathic cancer pain: Prevalence, severity, analgesics and impact from the European Palliative Care Research Collaborative computerised symptom assessment study. *Palliative Medicine*. 2012; **27**:714–21.

4. Paice JA. Pain. In Dahlin C, Coyne PJ, Ferrell BR, eds. *Advanced Practice Palliative Nursing*. New York: Oxford University Press, 2016, 219–32.

Chemotherapy-Induced Peripheral Neuropathy

Kimberly Chow

Clinical History

KS was a 46-year-old woman in her usual state of health when she began developing symptoms of heartburn and weight loss. She attributed these symptoms to stress from working a full-time job as an administrative assistant as well as caring for her three teenage children. As her symptoms persisted, KS also began noticing some discomfort with swallowing that prompted her to see her physician. She went for an endoscopy for further evaluation at which time she was found to have an esophageal stricture with a biopsy positive for squamous cell carcinoma. A CT scan of her chest, abdomen, and pelvis was performed for further workup and it revealed metastatic disease to the lung and retroperitoneal lymph nodes.

KS was seen by an oncologist who recommended systemic therapy, which he explained would be palliative in nature, with the hopes of stabilizing the disease, improving quality of life, and prolonging survival. Two weeks later, KS was started on a first-line chemotherapy regimen of fluorouracil, oxaliplatin, and leucovorin (FOLFOX). Shortly after beginning treatment, she began noticing a numbing sensation in her fingertips that progressively worsened to feelings of pins and needles. This caused a significant level of discomfort for KS, particularly since her job required her to work on the computer.

Follow-up scans at three months to assess her response to treatment showed that overall her disease remained stable, with a slight decrease in the lung metastases. KS was relieved and her oncologist recommended that she continue on with the current treatment regimen. She reported her symptoms of discomfort to her oncologist, who told her this may be a potential side effect of chemotherapy. He felt it would be best to still continue on with treatment and he prescribed a low dose of gabapentin 100 mg every eight hours for chemotherapy-induced peripheral neuropathy (CIPN).

As KS continued on with treatment, her neuropathy worsened and it began interfering with both her job and her ability to care for her family. At a subsequent visit, KS demanded that her chemotherapy regimen be discontinued due to uncontrolled pain. Her oncologist requested a same-day palliative care consult to offer better pain and symptom relief.

Examination

Her neurologic exam was grossly non-focal. She had full strength in all muscle groups bilaterally. There was decreased sensation in her fingertips to pinprick and her hands were cool to the touch.

Palliative Domains of Care

Physical Aspects of Care

KS described her pain mostly in her fingertips, although at times her entire hand felt painfully numb. Her fingertips constantly felt cold and they were sensitive to touch, which impaired her ability to cook, clean, type, and stay active. She found herself easily irritated by her husband and kids and she constantly felt overwhelmed at work. She stated, "My fingers feel like they're always asleep. And sometimes an electrical pain will just shoot through my fingers in the middle of the night." At best her pain was "6 out of 10"; at worst she rated her pain as "9 out of 10." She had been taking gabapentin 100 mg by mouth every eight hours for the past three weeks without any relief. She denied any adverse effects.

In addition to her neuropathic pain, KS also reported a low level of discomfort across her upper abdomen that she described as fullness and tenderness at times. She rated this pain as "4 out of 10" and it was exacerbated by eating and by lying flat.

Cultural and Social Aspects of Care

When asking KS how she would describe herself as a person, she stated that she very much identified with being a wife, a mother, and a highly independent career woman. She had worked for the same high-level executive for more than ten years and she prided herself on the success of her department. In her home life, KS attended all of her children's sporting events and she even practiced softball with her 13-year-old daughter. She stated, "If I can't be the person I've always been, then none of this is worth it to me."

Palliative Care Discussion

Neuropathic pain is classified as pain that arises from damage to the peripheral or central nervous system [1]. Neuropathic pain is often underdiagnosed and undertreated, with prevalence ranging between 19 and 40 percent in various studies [2, 3]. Patients often describe the sensation as burning, shooting, electrical, numbness, or tingling.

CIPN is a known acute and chronic side effect of various chemotherapeutic agents, including taxane and platinum derivatives [4]. Studies suggest the negative impact of CIPN on quality of life and functional ability for patients living with cancer [4, 5]. The management approach to CIPN includes first assessing the level of toxicity of treatment and whether the patient can safely continue on with therapy. For patients with disease response to the chemotherapeutic regimen and low to moderate levels of CIPN, a trial of pharmacologic and non-pharmacologic methods of pain relief is reasonable.

The majority of studies on pharmacologic management strategies have been focused primarily on non-CIPN such as diabetic neuropathy. The pathogenesis and symptomatology of CIPN is different from non-CIPN, which may lead to different treatment effects. However, given the limited definitive data on CIPN, it would be appropriate to use similar treatment algorithms [5]. Adjuvant analgesics such as antidepressants and antiepileptics continue to be the recommended first-line therapy in chronic neuropathic pain. Patients should be started on low doses and gradually titrated up to therapeutic effect with a trial of approximately four to six weeks at target dosing [1, 5, 6].

Opioids, including tramadol, have also demonstrated some efficacy in both CIPN and non-CIPN and are recommended as second- or third-line treatments of non-CIPN neuropathic pain. Early studies on non-pharmacologic therapies, including acupuncture, exercise, and neuro-stimulation, show some promising benefit and should be considered as part of the overall treatment plan [5].

Treatment Course

KS was able to continue on with treatment with close follow-up by the palliative care team. Her gabapentin was titrated up by 300 mg every four days [6] to reach a therapeutic dose of 900 mg by mouth every eight hours, which she felt offered drastic improvements in her pain control. For episodes of severe shooting pain, particularly at night, and for her visceral abdominal pain, likely from tumor involvement, KS was prescribed oxycodone on an as-needed basis. She had a short trial of duloxetine, which she self-discontinued due to feelings of dizziness.

As KS's disease eventually progressed, she was rotated off of FOLFOX and she enrolled in a clinical trial. Despite transitioning off of platinum-based therapy, she continued with low levels of chronic neuropathy in her hands and feet that remained controlled on adjuvant analgesics. She began developing worsening upper abdominal pain from tumor progression, which she found long-acting and fast-acting opioids to be the most effective in treating.

General Remarks

Pain has been reported in up to 60 percent of patients receiving active treatment for cancer [7]. The etiology of these pain reports includes pain from direct tumor involvement as well as pain from treatments such as chemotherapy, surgery, and radiation therapy. CIPN falls within this category and may offer a compelling reason to discontinue therapies that are otherwise working to control a patient's disease.

From the start of disease-targeted treatments, independent of the diagnosis, patients and their families should be educated on the potential side effects of treatment and what to expect. In KS's case, early education and a stepwise approach to her early complaints of CIPN could have minimized suffering and improved overall quality of life throughout her illness.

Suggested Reading

1. International Association for the Study of Pain (IASP). Diagnosis and classification of neuropathic pain. 2010. www.iasp-pain.org/PublicationsNews/NewsletterIssue .aspx?ItemNumber=2083. Accessed March 23, 2017.

2. Bennett MI, Rayment C, Hjermstad M, et al. Prevalence and aetiology of neuropathic pain in cancer patients: A systematic review. *Pain.* 2011;**153**:359–65.

3. Rayment C, Hjermstad MJ, Aass N, et al. Neuropathic cancer pain: Prevalence, severity, analgesics and impact from the European Palliative Care Research

Collaborative computerised symptom assessment study. *Palliative Medicine*. 2012;**27**:714–21.

4. Mols F, Beijers T, Vreugdenhil G, van de Poll-Franse L. Chemotherapy-induced peripheral neuropathy and its association with quality of life: A systematic review. *Support Care Cancer*. 2014;**22**: 2261–9.

5. Pachman DR, Watson JC, Lustberg MB, et al. Management options for established chemotherapy-induced peripheral neuropathy. *Support Care Cancer*. 2014;**22**:2281–95.

6. Paice JA. Pain. In Dahlin C, Coyne PJ, Ferrell BR, eds. *Advanced Practice Palliative Nursing*. New York: Oxford University Press, 2016, 219–32.

7. Paice JA. Pain at the end of life. In Ferrell BR, Coyle N, Paice J, eds. *Oxford Textbook of Palliative Nursing, 4th Edition*. New York: Oxford University Press. 2015, 135–53.

"Two Years May Be Too Far Away"

Kathryn Nevel and Alan Carver

Clinical History

A 58-year-old man with a history of right temporal lobe glioblastoma multiforme (GBM) is transferring care due to disease progression.

After discovery of a right temporal lobe mass 11 months prior, the patient was treated with standard therapy including gross total resection of the tumor, focused radiation, and concurrent temozolomide chemotherapy. He was stable following six cycles of adjuvant temozolomide when he developed precipitous onset of severe headaches, nausea, and vomiting. These symptoms prompted an emergency room evaluation at a local hospital, where he was found to have hydrocephalus. An MRI brain with and without contrast confirmed leptomeningeal spread of his malignancy (Figure 36.1). The patient underwent emergent ventriculoperitoneal shunt placement, with resolution of headaches, nausea, vomiting.

He presented to the neuro-oncology clinic two weeks after shunt placement for transfer of care. Per recommendations of the new neuro-oncologist, he started bevacizumab and lomustine for treatment of the GBM with leptomeningeal metastases.

At a follow-up visit six weeks later, a repeat MRI brain and spine was notable for stable leptomeningeal enhancement (Figures 36.2 and 36.3). There was no evidence of disease progression radiographically or clinically.

Figure 36.1 Axial T1 brain MRI with gadolinium shows hydrocephalus prior to the placement of a ventriculoperitoneal shunt

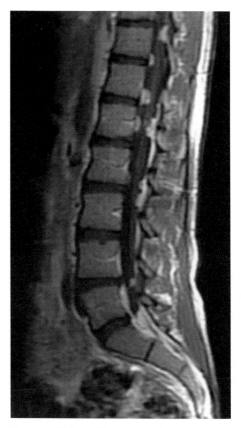

Figure 36.2 Sagittal lumbar spine MRI shows leptomeningeal deposits

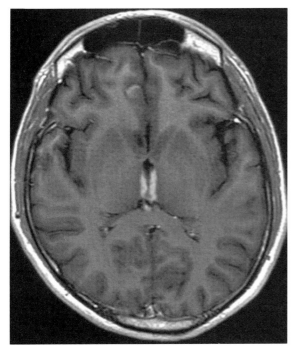

Figure 36.3 Axial T1 brain MRI with gadolinium reveals leptomeningeal enhancement in the third ventricle and in the right frontal paramedian sulcus

Examination

He was alert and oriented with a normal cognitive evaluation. Cranial nerves were notable for a left upper motor neuron (UMN) pattern facial droop, a mild left hemiparesis, and a mildly hemiparetic gait. Babinski sign was present bilaterally. The sensory exam was notable for signs of left-sided neglect. His exam at follow-up was stable compared to six weeks prior.

Palliative Domain of Care

Structure and Process of Care: Prognostic awareness

A conversation about prognosis was not held at the time of the initial consultation with the current treating neuro-oncologist, and it was unknown if prior discussions regarding prognosis had taken place.

At the end of the six-week follow-up visit, the patient and his wife said they were looking forward to going wedding dress shopping with their daughter. The patient and his daughter were notably close and he commented that he enjoyed participating in the wedding-planning activities. A date in Europe for the ceremony was set in two years. While the patient and his family were aware that he had a serious illness that may shorten his life span, there was no uncertainty expressed that the patient would be present at the wedding.

Palliative Care Discussion

The plan to attend his daughter's wedding in two years implied that he and his family may lack prognostic awareness of his condition. Given the median overall survival in patients with glioblastoma multiforme from time of diagnosis of leptomeningeal metastases is between three and a half to seven months, and patients with GBM on average survive 14–15 months, it seemed highly unlikely that the patient would be present at such an important family event two years into the future [1, 2].

A discussion with the patient, his wife, and daughter was held with the intent of obtaining a better grasp of their expectations, hopes, and understanding of his disease and treatment. While the patient and his wife understood that his diagnosis of glioblastoma may be associated with a shorter life expectancy, they did not express a clear understanding of his prognosis. On the contrary, they were under the impression that his current cancer-directed treatments had potential for cure, which is not uncommon among patients with advanced cancer [3]. During this discussion, they identified one personal goal of treatment: to feel well enough to attend his daughter's wedding in two years. The patient asked, "Do you think I will be alive in two years, doctor?"

This poignant question invited honest discussion between the physician, patient, and his wife regarding prognosis. The neuro-oncologist emphasized that while each patient is different, and there is always room for hope that the patient will live longer than expected, for patients with the same diagnosis life expectancy is usually measured in months and not years. He gently counseled that for important life goals, such as attending his daughter's wedding, alternate plans might be considered to assure that the entire family had the opportunity to celebrate together.

Clinical Course

Though a difficult conversation, the patient and his family expressed gratitude in having a better understanding of prognosis so that he could make plans to do what was important to him. Two months later the patient's daughter and fiancé held a small wedding ceremony at home among close family members and friends, which the patient attended. He received tumor-directed treatments for another seven months, and then transitioned to hospice care. He died nine months after the discovery of the leptomeningeal metastases.

General Remarks

Prognostic awareness in patients with progressive neurological diseases or advanced cancer is defined as an individual's understanding of his or her illness in terms of shortened life expectancy or outcome [4]. There are varying degrees of prognostic awareness – for example, in patients with glioblastoma multiforme this can range from understanding that the diagnosis shortens life span, to that it is an incurable cancer, to that the average life expectancy after diagnosis despite standard therapy is 14–15 months [5]. The presence of any degree of prognostic awareness in patients with malignant gliomas varies among small prospective studies, but with a trend toward increased prognostic awareness at the time of recurrence compared to after the initial diagnosis [6]. Providing patients with prognostic information while maintaining hope is usually viewed positively by patients. When patients have an understanding of their prognosis earlier in their disease process, they are given the opportunity to communicate their preferences before they are too ill to do so. They are also able to clarify their goals, particularly in the setting of a foreshortened life.

Earlier integration of palliative care is generally viewed favorably by patients, and has been shown to improve quality of life and prolong survival among patients with lung cancer [7]. The treating neuro-oncologist has an obligation to provide patients with evidence-based tumor-directed care in the form of chemotherapeutic agents, clinical trial options, and coordination of multidisciplinary care with surgery and radiation oncology, but also to provide comprehensive palliative care from the time of diagnosis [8].

For this patient, he was planning a very important life event two years in the future under the expectation that he would be alive and well enough to attend. Though he and his family never lost hope that he would be alive in two years to attend his daughter's wedding, after gaining a better prognostic awareness that it was more than likely he would not be, he walked his daughter down the aisle two months after hopeful, but honest discussions with the treating neuro-oncologist. The patient's family expressed their gratitude for finding a neuro-oncologist who considered it his obligation to not only do all that he could to treat the cancer, but also to help the patient and his family plan for an inevitably sad, yet more likely outcome.

Suggested Reading

1. Mandel JJ, Yust-Katz S, Cachia D, Wu J, Liu D, de Groot JF, Yung AW, Gilbert MR. Leptomeningeal dissemination in glioblastoma: An inspection of risk factors, treatment, and outcomes at a single institution. *J Neurooncol*. 2014 Dec;**120**(3):597–605.

2. De la Fuente MI, DeAngelis LM. The role of ventriculoperitoneal shunting in patients with supratentorial glioma. *Ann Clin Transl Neurol*. 2014 Jan;**1**(1):45–8.

3. Weeks JC, Catalano PJ, Cronin A, Finkelman MD, Mack JW, Keating NL, Schrag D. Patients' Expectations about effects of chemotherapy for advanced cancer. *N Engl J Med*. 2012 Oct;**367**(17):1616–25.

4. Diamond EL, Corner GW, De Rosa A, Breitbart W, Applebaum AJ. Prognostic awareness and communication of prognostic information in malignant glioma: A systematic review. *J Neurooncol*. 2014 Sep; **119**(2):227–34.

5. Stupp R, Mason WP, Van den Bent MJ, Weller M, Fisher B, Taphoorn MJ, Belanger K, Brandes AA, et al. Radiotherapy plus concomitant and adjuvant temozolomide for glioblastoma. *N Engl J Med*. 2005 Mar;**352**(10):987–96.

6. Davies E, Clarke C, Hopkins A. Malignant cerebral glioma – II: Perspectives of patients and relatives on the value of radiotherapy. *BMJ*. 1996 Dec;**313**(7971): 1512–16.

7. Temel JS, Greer JA, Muzikansky A, Gallagher ER, Admane S, Jackson VA, Dahlin CM, Blinderman CD, Jacobsen J, Pirl WF, Billings JA, Lynch TJ. Early palliative care for patients with metastatic non-small-cell lung cancer. *N Engl J Med*. 2010 Aug;**363**(8):733–42.

8. Thomas A, Carver A. Essential competencies in palliative medicine for neuro-oncologists. *Neuro-oncology Practice*. 2015 May;**2**(3):151–7.

Shifting the Goals of Care

Kathryn Nevel and Alan Carver

Clinical History

A 72-year-old woman with metastatic melanoma to the lung, liver, and left occipital lobe who had been treated with several regimens, currently on a BRAF inhibitor (dabrafineb) and methy ethyl kinase (MEK) inhibitor (trametinib), as well as congestive heart failure, presented with seizures.

Over the previous month, she developed worsening headaches, cognitive decline, gait instability, and falls. Though she had moved in with one of her daughters, she was performing most of her activities of daily living independently up until several days ago. On the day of admission, she had shaking movements of her left arm followed by her left leg with rapid generalization and loss of consciousness. The suspected seizure activity lasted about a minute before resolving without intervention, and emergency medical services (EMS) was called. She remained lethargic and was not back to baseline when EMS arrived. She then had further seizure-like activity of similar semiology, requiring intramuscular midazolam to abort the event, which lasted roughly four minutes. Upon arrival to the emergency department, she was stuporous, though her respiratory status was stable. She had never had a seizure before.

A head CT was performed that demonstrated a marked increase in the size of her known left occipital metastasis and seven new hemorrhagic brain metastases with surrounding edema (Figures 37.1 and 37.2). A CT chest/abdomen/pelvis also demonstrated marked progression of cancer with innumerable new multi-organ metastases. She was admitted to the neurology inpatient service for management of seizures and cerebral edema. Phenytoin and dexamethasone were started and she was placed on video EEG monitoring. Despite no evidence of continued seizures on the electroencephalogram (EEG), she remained deeply stuporous.

Examination

She was afebrile with a respiratory rate of 14 and oxygen saturation of 97 percent on 2 liters oxygen by nasal cannula. Mental status waxed and waned between stuporous and comatose states. She had a left upper motor neuron pattern facial droop, and when in a stuporous state she responded less vigorously to noxious stimuli on the left. She also had left-sided hyperreflexia, Babinski sign was present bilaterally. There was no evidence of suffering or distress.

Palliative Domain of Care

Structure and Process of Care – Determining goals of care

Shortly following admission, a meeting was held to delineate the goals of care, the patient's wishes with

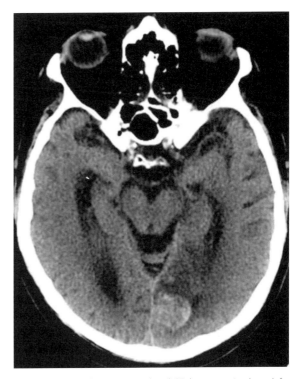

Figure 37.1 Axial non-contrast head CT demonstrating large left occipital hemorrhagic metastasis, which had increased in size from the last MRI two months prior

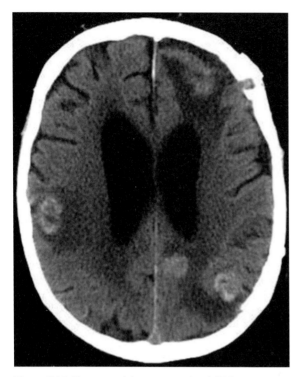

Figure 37.2 The same axial non-contrast head CT demonstrating four of seven hemorrhagic metastases with surrounding edema

regard to cardiopulmonary resuscitation (CPR), and to develop a mutually agreed upon treatment plan. The patient had stated in prior discussions with her treating physicians and daughters that she would not want to pursue additional cancer-directed therapies in the case of a relapse, and that she would want to focus on comfort and quality of life, which she defined as functioning independently. She had an advance care directive that identified her daughters as her health care surrogates, and she had expressed that she would not want to undergo CPR should she experience cardiac or pulmonary arrest. Her daughters confirmed that their mother would not want to receive CPR, and a Do-Not-Resuscitate (DNR) order was issued.

Palliative Care Discussion

Treatment options were discussed, including transitioning to comfort measures only, whole brain irradiation, stereotactic radiosurgery, further chemotherapy, or surgical intervention. While no clearly defined surgical target was identified, it was important to family that this option was explored. A multidisciplinary discussion was held among the neuro-oncologist, medical oncologist, radiation oncologist, and neurosurgeon to

discuss potential treatment options. The group provided a unified recommendation that further treatment was unlikely to be beneficial, and may be harmful, given her advanced metastatic cancer and poor functional status. In light of the patient's expressed wishes regarding treatment goals and her current condition with an increase in the number and size of metastases, her daughters felt it was in line with her wishes to not continue with cancer-directed treatments, and to focus on treating her seizures.

Once her goals of care were shifted to hospice, her daughters' focus shifted to taking her home safely, as the patient had told them in the past that she wanted to die at home. While they were hopeful they could take her home in order to honor her wishes, they were also concerned about their ability to care for her and that she would be "forgotten" by her medical team.

Essential barriers to providing competent palliative care have been identified as:

1) Physician misrepresenting palliative care as only equivalent to hospice care
2) Lack of competency among neuro-oncologists in the principles of palliative medicine
3) Patient underreporting symptoms due to fear of their significance
4) The "culture of cure" that many neuro-oncologists work in and many patients with brain tumors seek their care in, with its inherent focus upon the disease versus the patient with the disease [1].

Hospital Course

Video EEG was discontinued, as were lab draws, medications, and other interventions that were no longer consistent with the goals of care. After discussing with family that intravenous hydration may prolong quantity, but not necessarily improve her quality of life, the family elected to discontinue IV fluids as well. The outpatient oncologists reassured the daughters that the medical team would continue to care for their mother throughout the duration of her life – despite a change in goals of care. The patient was discharged home with hospice 12 days after hospital admission.

General Remarks

The end-of-life phase in patients with cancer is defined as when a patient has progressive cancer in the setting of clinical deterioration, and can no longer receive tumor-directed therapy. In patients who are at the end of life, the treating physicians must carefully weigh the potential risks and benefits of any intervention with the family. After discussing prognosis and pros and cons of possible further interventions, the patient's daughters were unanimous in their request to shift the goals of care to a focus upon symptom management only, which they felt was congruent with their mother's previously expressed wishes. After her goals of care were shifted, the daughters' main concerns were non-abandonment by her treating physicians and prevention of clinical seizures.

Seizures are commonly encountered in patients with brain tumors [2], and they can be challenging to manage effectively at the end of life in the setting of dysphagia or a depressed level of consciousness. The treatment of seizures at the end of life can include buccal administration of benzodiazepines, intranasal midazolam, or intramuscular phenobarbital [3, 4]. If needed, IV formulations can be continued in the hospital, hospice facility, and occasionally in the home if nursing care is coordinated.

For patients with a poor prognosis for survival, particularly those with brain tumors who may be unable to communicate late in their illness, it is important for the neuro-oncologist to discuss preferences for end-of-life care early in the disease course [5]. Ensuring a dignified death requires that the physician minimize a patient's symptoms, maximize a patient's function, and if possible, enable a person to die in their pre-identified preferred surroundings [6, 7]. A general approach to caring for patients with neurologic disorders at or near the end of life is outlined in Table 37.1.

Despite the shift in goals of care, the patient and family continued to be supported by the medical team – by managing symptoms, reassuring non-abandonment, and providing education and resources so family could care for the patient in her home. With these support systems in place, they took her home with hospice care, where she died peacefully five days after discharge. The treating neuro-oncologist fulfilled an emerging practice standard by demonstrating competency in palliative care in meeting the needs of his patient with brain metastases nearing the end of life.

Suggested Reading

1. Thomas AA, Carver A. Essential competencies in palliative medicine for neuro-oncologists. *Neuro-Oncology Practice*, 2015; **0**: 1–7.

2. Gofton TE, Graber J, Carver A. Identifying the palliative care needs of patients living with cerebral tumors and

Table 37.1 Palliative Care in Patients with Untreatable Neuro-Oncologic Disease [7]

1. Assure patients and their loved ones that even though the cancer is no longer being treated, that the patient and his/her symptoms will always be treated (assure non-abandonment)

2. Ask patients what they are most afraid of and address these concerns honestly. If patients are unable to participate in discussions due to depressed level of consciousness, confusion, or aphasia, ask patients' family members and friends

3. Provide symptom management—including but not limited to seizures, pain, nausea, dyspnea, terminal secretions. Ensure that treatment can still be administered in the case of progressive dysphagia by providing buccal, intranasal, and/or rectal formulations of necessary medications

4. Even if seizures have not occurred previously in a patient with intracranial tumor(s), provide a prescription for an as-needed benzodiazepine, in case a seizure should occur so the patient can be given an abortive medication quickly

5. Avoid reduction of steroid dosing unless necessary, as steroids may be providing symptom relief

6. Clarify a patients' health care proxy, if not already done

7. Provide Support to the family and friends of the patient

metastases: A retrospective analysis. *J Neurooncol.* 2012 July;**108**(3):527–34.

3. Pace A, Villani V, Di Lorenzo C, Guariglia L, Maschio M, Pompili A, Carapella CM. Epilepsy in the end-of-life phase in patients with high-grade gliomas. *J NEurooncol.* 2013 Jan;**111**(1):83–6.

4. Sizoo EM, Koekkoek JA, Postma TJ, Heimans JJ, Pasman HR, Deliens L, Taphoorn MJ, Rijneveld JC. Seizures in patients with high-grade glioma: A serious challenge in the end of life. *BMJ Support Palliat Care.* 2014 Mar;**4**(1):77–80.

5. Sizoo EM, Taphoorn MJ, Uitdehaag B, Heimans JJ, Deliens L, Reijneveld JC, Pasman HR. The end-of-life phase of high-grade glioma patients: Dying with dignity? *Oncologist.* 2013 Jan;**18**(2):198–203.

6. Chochinov HM, Hack T, Hassard T, Kristjanson LJ, McClement S, Harlos M. Dignity in the terminally ill: A cross-sectional, cohort study. *Lancet.* 2002 Dec;**360** (9350):2026–30.

7. Carver AC, Foley MF. Symptom assessment and management. *Neurology Clinics: Palliative Care.* Eds. AC Carver, KM Foley. Philadelphia, PA: W. B. Saunders, 2001. 940.

Management of Seizures in Patients with Glioma from Diagnosis through the End of Life

Kristen Chasteen, and Tobias Walbert

Clinical History

A 48-year-old woman who had been in good health experienced a witnessed seizure and was brought to the emergency department. Magnetic resonance imaging (MRI) revealed a right frontal enhancing lesion with features concerning for a high-grade glioma (Figure 38.1A). She underwent surgical resection and pathology was consistent with a WHO grade IV glioblastoma (Figure 38.1B). She received adjuvant radiation and temozolomide. She continued to show progression on MRI and she underwent three more craniotomies with resections (Figure 38.1C). She enrolled in a clinical trial, receiving multiple rounds of chemotherapy for approximately two years. After this period, she was noted to be stable and chemotherapy was discontinued. One year later, a follow-up MRI revealed progression of disease and chemotherapy was restarted. Despite chemotherapy, her disease

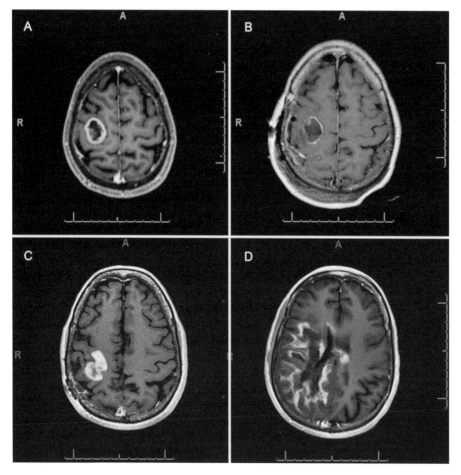

Figure 38.1 A. Patient presents with right frontal lesion. B. MRI showing the lesion after the first resection. C. MRI showing further progression. D. The final MRI prior to death showing extensive disease progression

continued to progress over the next two years (Figure 38.1D).

Palliative Domain of Care

Physical Aspects of Care – Seizures

Her clinical course was complicated by recurrent seizures. She was immediately started on levetiracetam 500 mg twice per day following her initial presentation with a generalized tonic-clonic seizure. She did well for two months, but then continued to have breakthrough seizures and her levetiracetam was increased in steps up to a total of 2,000 mg twice per day. The patient was compliant with her antiseizure medications, but eventually lacosamide was added. She had no seizures for another four years, but then again began having breakthrough seizures and phenytoin was added and titrated. She did well on this regimen until about six years following her initial diagnosis. Over a two-month period, she noticed a general functional and cognitive decline. Her MRI showed progressive disease (Figure 38.1C). She also began having left-sided weakness, which eventually caused her to become bedbound, and she had increased episodes of confusion as well as an overall decline in her appetite and oral intake. Her seizure activity increased, with reports of up to 10 seizures per day and she was found, on serial lab exams, to have sub-therapeutic total phenytoin as well as free phenytoin levels. Her phenytoin dose was subsequently increased. She did not have any further clinical seizures following these medication adjustments, but her functional status, MRI (Figure 38.1D), and overall clinical condition continued to decline.

Examination

She was alert and oriented to person and intermittently to place. She did not frequently participate in conversations. She had significant bilateral weakness in both upper and lower extremities.

Clinical Course

After discussion with her about the status of her disease and her goals for care, the primary neuro-oncology team made the recommendation for hospice enrollment. At time of admission to hospice, she was still taking pills by mouth, but was beginning to have symptoms of dysphagia, having problems with swallowing pills as well as with her regular diet. In hospice care, she was switched from the tablet form of medications to liquid forms to help with swallowing in the setting of increasing dysphagia. She was able to continue all of her seizure medications for a brief period of time after hospice enrollment, and initially she did well with this regimen. She had an order for lorazepam 2 mg subcutaneously as needed for seizures lasting longer than five minutes. Over the days preceding her death, she became increasingly confused and withdrawn, and she began to decline all meals. One day prior to her death, she had a seizure and was given the 2 mg subcutaneous lorazepam and the seizure stopped. That same day, she lost the ability to swallow any of the medications, including liquid formulations. She was initiated on therapy with 1 mg lorazepam subcutaneously scheduled every six hours for seizure prophylaxis with breakthrough lorazepam as needed for seizures. Maintaining alertness was no longer possible given the progression of her disease and the sedating side effects of lorazepam were not a concern. Subcutaneous access was obtained and allowed for easier administration than the sublingual route. She did not have any further seizures prior to her death.

General Remarks

How Common Are Seizures in Glioma Patients?

Epileptic seizures are common in patients with glioma and they occur more frequently in patients with low-grade tumors (60–80 percent) compared with WHO IV glioblastoma and anaplastic glioma (29–46 percent). Seizures are common at the time of diagnosis of a brain tumor and are the first presenting symptom in about 40 percent of patients. These patients remain at a higher increased risk for recurrent seizures despite treatment with anti-epileptic drugs (AEDs) [1]. Seizures are also common at the end of life, with about 30 percent of patients with glioma experiencing a seizure during the last week of life [2]. In this patient with a history of seizures, the hospice team correctly recognized that she was at risk of seizures at the end of life. However, seizures are also common in the last week of life for glioma patients without any seizure history [2]. A plan for seizure management needs to be a part of end-of-life care and counseling for all glioma patients.

How Should Seizures Be Treated in Patients with Glioma from the Time of Diagnosis?

Initiation of long-term treatment with an AED should be strongly considered after the first seizure in a patient with glioma given the increased risk of seizure recurrence in this population. Patients with low-grade glioma are at higher risk for seizures than patients with high-grade glioma. Primary anti-epileptic prophylaxis for glioma patients is currently not recommended for patients that have never had a seizure [3]. The pharmacokinetic interactions with anti-cancer therapies and other drugs should be considered when selecting an appropriate AED for treatment initiation. A number of older AEDs such as phenobarbital, phenytoin, primidone, carbamazepine, and oxcarbazepine induce the cytochrome 450 (CYP450)-dependent hepatic enzymes and influence the metabolism and efficacy of many commonly used cytotoxic agents as well as dexamethasone. Newer AEDs such as levetiracetam, lacosamide, and zonisamide don't influence CYP450 and have a much lower risk of drug–drug interactions. In the setting of brain tumor patients undergoing treatment, levetiracetam is the most studied newer-generation AED that is generically available and has limited side effects. Levetiracetam is the appropriate first-line treatment in glioma patients [1].

How Should Seizures Be Managed at the End of Life in Patients with Glioma?

Treatment of seizures becomes more difficult near the end of life as many patients with brain tumors lose the ability to take their normal AEDs due to somnolence or other swallowing difficulties [2]. Stopping AEDs could lead to higher risk of seizures in the last days of life, which may be very distressing to patients and families [2]. Seizures at the end of life could also cause families to call emergency medical services, resulting in an unwanted emergency department visit and hospital admission. Careful planning and proactive education for patients and families are necessary to prevent and to treat seizures at the end of life in the home setting. A hospice team would likely provide the best support for seizure and other end-of-life symptom management in the home setting. This patient was in a hospice residential care center with 24-hour nursing support, which is another good option depending on patient preferences and availability of support at home.

There is minimal empirical evidence to guide seizure prevention and management in patients near death. Most of the recommendations come from case reports and expert opinion. It is recommended that AEDs are continued for as long as possible in patients with glioma and a prior seizure history and that all patients with glioma have an as-needed medication that is available to treat possible seizures at the end of life [4]. Extended-release formulations may need to be changed to immediate release tablets or oral suspensions if patients begin to have trouble swallowing pills whole. For patients who become unable to swallow, administration of AEDs through the nasal, buccal, sublingual, intravenous (IV), subcutaneous (SC), and rectal routes may be considered [5–7]. The intramuscular route is generally avoided at the end of life given increased pain compared to other options. Most AEDs can be given IV, however, IV access is often difficult in the home setting and can be uncomfortable for patients at the end of life. Successful subcutaneous administration of levetiracetam has been described in multiple case reports [8, 9] and lacosamide in one case report [10], although neither is licensed for administration by that route. Given the lower risk of sedation compared to alternatives, subcutaneous levetiracetam and lacosamide are options to consider in patients who lose the ability to swallow but still desire to be as alert as possible. Cost may be a barrier to use in the hospice setting. Use of subcutaneous phenobarbital has also been described as effective for prevention and treatment of seizures at the end of life and could be considered for patients where additional sedation is not a concern [5]. Use of scheduled buccal clonazepam has been described for prevention of seizures at the end of life in patients with glioma [6] and scheduled sublingual lorazepam could also be considered. Rectal administration of AEDs can be considered; however, it may not be an acceptable route for patients and caregivers. Additionally, bioavailability with rectal administration may not be equivalent to oral dosing for some medications. There is evidence that carbamazepine, lamotrigine, levetiracetam, phenobarbital, topiramate, and valproate can be administered rectally. Limited evidence indicates that rectal administration is not effective for clonazepam, felbamate, gabapentin, lorazepam, midazolam, oxcarbazepine, or phenytoin [6].

Non-IV options for treatment of acute seizures at the end of life include intranasal, buccal, or subcutaneous midazolam, sublingual or subcutaneous lorazepam, and rectal diazepam. The efficacy of rectal diazepam was similar to intra-nasal or buccal midazolam; however, caregivers preferred the buccal or intra-nasal routes [7]. Intra-nasal administration may be easier than buccal or sublingual administration without patient cooperation during an acute seizure. Caregivers may also have more discomfort with administering subcutaneous medications in the home setting.

Suggested Reading

1. Walbert T, Chasteen K. Palliative and supportive care for glioma patients. *Cancer Treat Res.* 2015;**163**:171–84.

2. Sizoo EM, Koekkoek JAF, Postma TJ, et al. Seizures in patients with high grade glioma: A serious challenge in the end-of-life phase. *BMJ Support Palliative Care*, 2013; 0:1–4.

3. Glantz MJ, Cole BF, Forsyth PA, et al. Practice parameter: Anticonvulsant prophylaxis in patients with newly diagnosed brain tumors. Report of the Quality Standards Subcommittee of the American Academy of Neurology. *Neurology.* 2000;**54**:1886–93.

4. Fritz L, Dirven L, Reijneveld JC, et al. Advance care planning in glioblastoma patients. *Cancers.* 2016;**8**:11.

5. Rémi C, Zwanzig V, Feddersen B. Subcutaneous use of lacosamide. *J Pain Symptom Management.* 2016;**51**:e2–4.

6. Koekkoek J, Postman T, Heimans J, et al. Antiepileptic drug treatment in the end-of-life phase of glioma patients: A feasibility study. *Support Care Cancer.* 2016; **24**:1633–8.

7. Anderson GD, Saneto RP. Current oral and non-oral routes of anti-epileptic drug delivery. *Advanced Drug Delivery Rev.* 2012;**64**:911–18.

8. Rémi C, Lorenzl S. Continuous subcutaneous use of levetiracetam: A retrospective review of tolerability and clinical effects. *J Pain Palliative Care Pharmacother.* 2014;**28**(4):371–7.

9. Lopez-Saca J, Vaquero J, Larumbe A, et al. Repeated use of subcutaneous levetiracetam in a palliative care patient. *J Pain Symptom Management.* 2013;**45**(5): e7–8.

10. Jain P, Sharma S, Dua T, et al. Efficacy and safety of anti-epileptic drugs in patients with active convulsive seizures when no IV access is available: Systematic review and meta-analysis. *Epilepsy Res.* 2016;**122**: 47–55.

The Burden of Health Care Surrogacy in the Absence of Instruction

Ugur Sener and Maisha T. Robinson

Clinical History

An 88-year-old right-handed woman with a history of breast cancer and having undergone surgery and chemotherapy nine years prior, coronary artery disease, and paroxysmal atrial fibrillation presented to the neurology clinic for evaluation of new neurologic symptoms. She had developed mild left-sided weakness with family members describing occasional drooling from the left side of the mouth and difficulty with use of her left upper extremity. She was slurring her words and she appeared confused to her family members, hitting doors and furniture while ambulating through her house.

Magnetic resonance imaging (MRI) of the brain demonstrated multicentric mass lesions with heterogeneous enhancement primarily involving the right parietal, temporal, and occipital lobes associated with significant vasogenic edema (Figure 39.1). The right temporal mass lesion had an area of central necrosis. A biopsy was performed and histological analysis revealed a high-grade glial neoplasm consistent with glioblastoma multiforme (GBM). Isocitrate dehydrogenase 1 (IDH1) mutation was not detected. O(6)-methylguanine-DNA methyltransferase (MGMT) promoter methylation was absent.

Upon diagnosis of GBM, she was started on dexamethasone, which improved her left-sided weakness and dysarthria. Prognosis was reviewed with her and with her family members. Neurology and radiation-oncology consultants indicated a median survival of three to six months for untreated GBM. Radiation therapy alone, chemotherapy with temozolomide alone, and combined chemoradiation were discussed as treatment options. Family declined radiation therapy due to concerns regarding side effects such as fatigue, cognitive decline, and alopecia. The tentative plan was made to start chemotherapy with temozolomide.

Examination

She was afebrile, hypertensive (154/93), and had a normal heart rate (68 beats per minute). She was awake, alert, and oriented except to the floor of the building she was visiting. She had normal speech and language function. Left homonymous hemianopia and mild left lower facial weakness were noted with the remainder of cranial nerve function being normal. Parietal drift was present in the left arm. Fine motor movements of the left foot were subtly abnormal. Gait evaluation was significant for

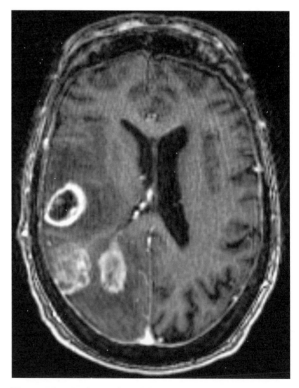

Figure 39.1 Axial T1 with gadolinium MRI brain indicating multicentric mass lesion with vasogenic edema involving the right temporal, parietal, and occipital lobes. Area of central necrosis is evident within the left temporal mass lesion.

a slightly wide-based gait with diminished stride length.

Palliative Domain of Care

Ethical and Legal Aspects of Care

She had a health care surrogate form, which had been signed three years prior to her diagnosis of GBM. This document designated her son as her surrogate decision maker in the event that she became incapacitated and unable to make medical decisions. The document did not specify her wishes regarding life-prolonging measures such as mechanical ventilation, artificial nutrition, or hydration. She had not extensively discussed these topics with her family members and her preferences were unknown.

Palliative Care Discussion

She had begun the advance care planning process by designating her son as the person who would assist with making medical decisions if she lacked the capacity to do so. However, she had neither documented nor discussed with her son or with her treating physicians what her preferences were with regard to life-prolonging care, despite having had another serious medical condition nine years prior to her new diagnosis.

In the absence of this information, her health care surrogate would be tasked with extrapolating his knowledge of what she would deem as a good quality of life, understanding the current clinical situation, and working with the medical teams to align the available treatment options with her presumed goals of care. This can be a challenging role for family members and other designated decision makers, particularly in the absence of prior guidance from the patient [1].

Clinical Course

Laboratory studies were obtained one day after her neurology clinic consultation in anticipation of the initiation of temozolomide chemotherapy. She was found to have thrombocytopenia with a platelet count at 74,000. Chemotherapy was held. Repeat laboratory evaluation one week later indicated persistent thrombocytopenia. The decision was made to hold temozolomide and to discuss further treatment options in clinic. Before the clinic appointment could take place, she presented to the emergency department with malaise, intermittent confusion, and hypertension.

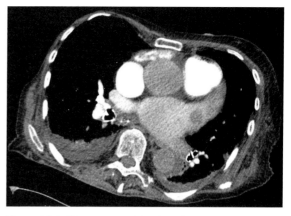

Figure 39.2 CT angiogram of the chest demonstrating a filling defect in the left atrial appendage, consistent with a left atrial appendage thrombus

Shortly after her hospital admission, she had a generalized tonic clonic seizure and she became somnolent. She was started on levetiracetam, but she continued to have intermittent rhythmic movements of the right hand and face. She was evaluated with an electroencephalogram (EEG), which showed periodic lateralized epileptiform discharges. She was started on phenytoin and later on lacosamide.

She developed right lower extremity swelling with identification of a deep venous thrombosis on ultrasound imaging. She developed atrial fibrillation with rapid ventricular response with computed tomography (CT) angiogram indicating a left atrial appendage thrombus (Figure 39.2). She was started on heparin for anticoagulation.

She remained somnolent with one-word responses to questions and she had difficulty following commands for three days. During this time, she was given intravenous fluids for hydration. Artificial nutrition was discussed with family members and a decision was made to place a nasogastric tube to provide nutrition. Her cognitive status subsequently improved and she removed her nasogastric tube on her own, on the same day it was placed. She became more alert and conversant by the fifth day of hospitalization. The inpatient neurology and radiation oncology teams, along with the patient, her son, and her daughter, discussed prognosis, treatment options, and goals of care in detail. She ultimately came to the conclusion that she did not want life-prolonging measures without improving her quality of life. Artificial nutrition was not reattempted. Intravenous hydration was discontinued.

Family members understood that without treatment, the life expectancy for GBM would be in the order of weeks, shorter in light of complications such as seizures and venous thrombosis. She was enrolled in hospice and discharged to an inpatient hospice facility. She passed away four days later.

General Remarks

GBM is the most common malignant brain tumor and it carries a poor prognosis with median survival of 14 months [2]. Maximal safe surgical resection followed by adjuvant radiotherapy plus concomitant and adjuvant temozolomide chemotherapy is currently considered the standard of care for GBM [3, 4]. Advanced age is thought to be an unfavorable prognostic factor with the optimum treatment regimen for elderly patients yet to be determined [3]. In general, presence of an IDH1 mutation has been associated with a better prognosis [5]. MGMT promoter methylation has also been associated with better progression free and overall survival in patients with GBM [6]. In this case, her tumor was IDH1 wildtype and lacked MGMT promoter methylation.

During the short course of disease, GBM can result in significant functional impairment and decline in quality of life [2, 7]. Seizures, headaches, mood symptoms, nausea, cognitive decline, fatigue, and focal neurologic deficits are among the complications of GBM [2, 7]. Early referral to palliative care can aid with management of these symptoms while facilitating goals-of-care discussions to ensure care received is in line with the patient's wishes.

In this case, she had a left homonymous hemianopia at the time of diagnosis, making it difficult for her to live independently. She moved in with her son to have assistance with activities of daily living. Over time, she also adapted to her visual field deficit and improved her ability to ambulate on her own. A home health evaluation could have been of further help in this regard, helping the family make household modifications to prevent falls and make it easier to maintain ambulatory status.

She could have also benefited from an earlier discussion of care at the end of life. She had a rapid deterioration in her cognitive status, which precluded her from making decisions regarding hydration and artificial nutrition. She was given intravenous hydration and she underwent placement of a nasogastric tube. Although she had a health care surrogate form designating her son as her health care surrogate, the topics of nutrition and hydration had not been explicitly discussed and her wishes were unknown at the time of her initial hospitalization. Given her self-removal of her nasogastric tube and her decline of hydration and nutrition later during her hospital stay, she may not have wanted these measures to be undertaken in the first place.

Her clinical course was complicated by the development of seizures, venous thrombosis, and atrial fibrillation with rapid ventricular response. She underwent multiple diagnostic studies, including prolonged EEG monitoring, venous ultrasound imaging, and CT angiogram. Her seizures remained difficult to control, eventually requiring the use of three antiseizure medications. She was treated with an intravenous anticoagulant. She was again unable to indicate whether she wanted to undergo these diagnostic studies or to receive the treatments administered. She may have preferred symptomatic management and comfort measures rather than diagnostic testing and additional treatments. She may have elected earlier enrollment in hospice with care delivered in the home setting rather than at a hospital.

Ultimately, her cognition improved and she could directly participate in the medical decision-making process. She discussed her condition with her family members and she elected to focus on comfort measures. She was transitioned to an inpatient hospice setting where she spent her final days with her children. In this case, palliative care consultation at the time of GBM diagnosis could have facilitated an earlier and more comprehensive discussion of end-of-life measures, perhaps leading to a smoother transition to hospice care. In the setting of a malignant central nervous system neoplasm, the possibility of a rapid cognitive deterioration as that which occurred for this patient underscores the need for having end-of-life discussions early and preparing an advance directive that reflects the patient's goals of care.

Suggested Reading

1. Vig E, Starks H, Taylor J, Hopley E, Fryer K. Surviving surrogate decision-making: What helps and hampers the experience of making medical decisions for others. *J Gen Intern Med.* 2007 Sep;22(9):1274–9.

2. Lin E, Rosenthal M, Le B, Eastman P. Neuro-oncology and palliative care: A challenging interface. *Neuro-oncology.* 2012;**14**:iv3–iv7.

3. Tanaka S, Meyer FB, Buckner JC, Uhm JH, Yan ES, Parney IF. Presentation, management, and outcome of

newly diagnosed glioblastoma in elderly patients. *J Neurosurg.* 2013;**118**:786–98.

4. Stupp R, Mason W, Van den Bent M, Weller M, Fisher B, Taphoorn M, Belanger K, Brandes A, Marosi C, Bogdahn U, Curschmann J, Janzer R, Ludwin S, Gorlia T, Allgeier A, Lacombe D, Cairncross G, Eisenhauer E, Mirimanoff R. Radiotherapy plus concomitant and adjuvant temozolomide for glioblastoma. *N Engl J Med.* 2005;**352**: 987–96.

5. Sanson M, Marie Y, Paris S, Idbaih A, Laffaire J, Ducray F, El Hallani S, Boisselier B, Mokhtari K, Hoang-Xuan K, Delattre JY. Isocitrate Dehydrogenase 1 Codon 132 mutation is an important prognostic biomarker in gliomas. *J Clin Oncol.* 2009;**27**(25): 4150–4.

6. Zhang K, Wang XQ, Zhou B, Zhang L. The prognostic value of MGMT promoter methylation in Glioblastoma multiforme: A meta-analysis. *Familial Cancer.* 2013;**12**: 449–58.

7. Hemminger LE, Pittman C, David NK, and Mohile NA. Palliative and end-of-life care in glioblastoma: Defining and measuring opportunities to improve care. *Neurooncol Pract.* 2016;npw022.

"But My Brother Should Be Treated"

Ugur Sener and Maisha T. Robinson

Clinical History

A 70-year-old man with a history of hypertension, hyperlipidemia, fibromyalgia, and melanoma excised six years ago presented to the neurology clinic for evaluation of a left cerebral mass. He had developed imbalance three months prior, which was initially attributed to a vestibulopathy. He underwent physical and occupational therapy for gait and balance training. When his symptoms failed to improve, magnetic resonance imaging (MRI) of the brain was obtained, which showed a large left cingulate gyrus lesion concerning for metastasis (Figure 40.1). Smaller left frontal, left parietal opercular, and left lentiform nucleus lesions were also identified (Figure 40.2). Computed tomography (CT) of the chest, abdomen, and pelvis was obtained, which identified a 1.6 cm nodule in the right upper lobe. The nodule was biopsied with immunohistochemical stains demonstrating neoplastic cells positive for S-100, Melan A, focal HMB45, MITF, and E-Cadherin, consistent with a diagnosis of metastatic malignant melanoma.

Upon identification of metastatic brain lesions, he was started on dexamethasone, which led to some improvement in his balance. However, he needed to

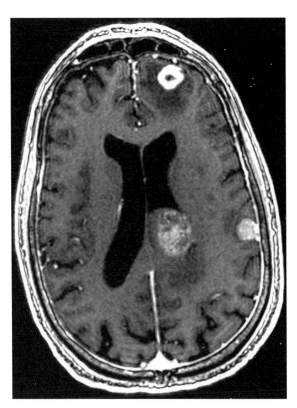

Figure 40.1 MRI brain T1 post-contrast imaging showing a large left cingulate gyrus, left frontal, and a left parietal opercular mass lesion concerning for metastasis

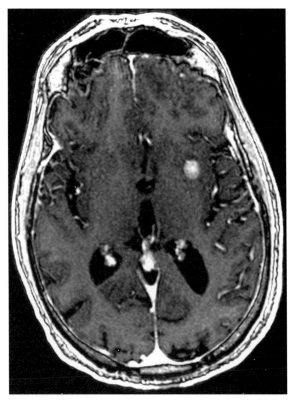

Figure 40.2 MRI brain T1 post-gadolinium image showing a left lentiform nucleus mass lesion

hold on to furniture in his house to ambulate. He had sustained three falls over a three-month period. He also described one episode of transient right hemi-sensory loss and incoordination. Outside pathology slides were requested for review with subsequent confirmation of the metastatic melanoma diagnosis. After consultation with radiation oncology, a plan was made to start systemic chemotherapy and to perform stereotactic radiosurgery on the brain metastases.

Examination

He was afebrile, hypertensive (148/72), and bradycardic (56 beats per minute). He was awake, alert, and oriented with normal language function. His speech was mildly dysarthric. He had mild right lower facial weakness with the remainder of the cranial nerve examination being normal. The motor examination revealed mild right-sided weakness and his gait evaluation was significant for a wide-based ataxic gait. He was unable to tandem walk.

Palliative Domain of Care

Ethical and Legal Aspects of Care

He had an advance directive, which was completed shortly after his consultation in neurology and radiation oncology clinics. The document designated his niece as his surrogate decision maker. He was not married, did not have any children, and was estranged from his two brothers. The directive stated that he would not want any life-prolonging measures such as mechanical ventilation, blood transfusion, artificial nutrition, or hydration if he had a terminal condition, an end-stage condition, or if he were in a persistent vegetative state and if physicians indicated that there was no reasonable chance of recovery. The advance directive also indicated that he did not wish to receive chemotherapy or radiation in the absence of substantial medical probability of improvement.

Palliative Care Discussion

Patients with serious or advanced medical conditions, particularly those that may progress to involve cognitive decline, should engage in advance care planning discussions soon after their diagnosis. This usually entails a series of conversations regarding their goals of care, what constitutes a good quality of life for them, and what type of medical care they want when they are at the end of their lives. As part of this discussion, patients are asked to identify who they would want to make medical decisions for them if they are unable to make them independently. They are also encouraged to document their preferences in an advance directive [1].

He clearly indicated that if he became mentally incapacitated and if he were unable to direct his medical care, then his niece would assist with determining what interventions, treatments, or procedures he should undergo that would align with his goals of care. He also documented that he did not want his life prolonged if there was no reasonable chance of improvement in his overall condition. Palliative care teams may be involved in situations in which there are complex family dynamics or family members have differing opinions regarding treatment options [2]. The interdisciplinary team can participate in family meetings and the various team members can provide spiritual, social, and psychological support to the patient and to the family members during the course of illness.

Hospital Course

Five days after the initial clinic evaluation, he was driving when he suddenly developed worsening right-sided weakness and dysarthria. Emergency department evaluation with a non-contrast CT of the head revealed a left basal ganglia intraparenchymal hemorrhage, at the location of the known left lentiform nucleus metastatic lesion (Figure 40.3). He was hospitalized in the intensive care unit with a dense right hemiparesis and worsened dysarthria. Language function became impaired secondary to an expressive aphasia. During his hospital course, he was disoriented to time and place and he was intermittently agitated.

Radiation oncology had originally planned stereotactic radiosurgery for the four metastatic brain lesions. However, due to interval development of intraparenchymal hemorrhage, the treatment field could no longer be fully visualized. As such, the recommendation was made for whole-brain radiation. After explanation of the risks and benefits, he declined radiation therapy.

The patient's twin brother arrived at the hospital and he initially requested that the patient begin whole-brain radiation, a treatment that was inconsistent with the patient's expressed goals of care. Due to the development of expressive aphasia and disorientation, communication with the patient was limited. A psychiatry consultation was therefore requested

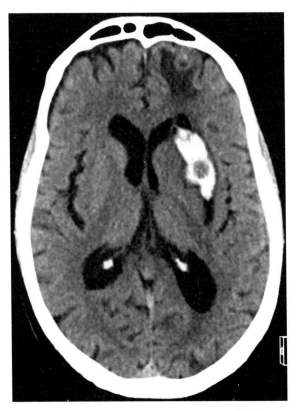

Figure 40.3 CT head non-contrast image showing left basal ganglia intraparenchymal hemorrhage at the location of previously identified left lentiform nucleus mass lesion

for a capacity evaluation. The patient said no when asked if he wanted to undergo radiation therapy. When asked if he understood the consequences, he stated, "I die." The psychiatry team reiterated the proposed treatment plan, including the risks and benefits. The patient again stated that he did not wish to undergo any radiation therapy or chemotherapy. The questions were repeated for a third time with the patient consistently declining radiation therapy. He communicated that he did not want to prolong his life under the present circumstances. With the permission of the patient, his twin brother was included in the discussion and he witnessed the patient articulate his desired plan of care firsthand. Although it was not necessary to involve his twin brother in the decision-making process as he was not his health care surrogate, the inclusion of all present family members allowed them to understand – and ultimately support – the patient's desired treatment plan.

The patient's stated wishes were in line with his advance directive as well as his prior discussions with his niece. It was concluded that he had capacity to refuse medical treatment. He was enrolled in hospice and discharged to an inpatient hospice facility. He passed away one week later.

General Remarks

Brain metastases are estimated to occur in 10–30 percent of cancer patients [3]. As a group, brain metastases represent the most common type of intracranial neoplasm, with numbers exceeding primary central nervous system (CNS) malignancies [4]. Melanoma is the third most common type of cancer to involve the brain, after lung and breast tumors [5]. In melanoma, brain metastases carry a very poor prognosis with an estimated median survival of 4.7 months after diagnosis [5].

Due to mass effect and vasogenic edema, brain metastases can lead to significant morbidity, including focal neurologic deficits and seizures. Metastatic melanoma has also been recognized as a brain lesion that is particularly prone to intracerebral hemorrhage, which can lead to sudden severe neurologic decline with development of motor, sensory, language, or visual deficits [6]. Patients are at risk of developing cognitive decline and fatigue with treatments aimed at managing symptoms [7]. Palliative care for patients with metastatic brain tumors remains challenging, requiring a multidisciplinary approach that maximizes supportive measures while avoiding potentially harmful treatments [7].

This case highlights the degree of physical impairment that can occur in the setting of metastatic melanoma. His metastatic brain tumors initially manifested as gait difficulty and imbalance. He sustained three falls and he had difficulty navigating through his house. Early involvement of palliative care at the time of diagnosis can help with management of these symptoms. Referral to physical and occupational therapy can lead to an improvement in functional status and gait-assist devices such as walkers can improve safety and prevent falls while helping patients maintain their independence for as long as possible.

Metastatic melanoma also carries the potential for sudden neurologic decline with the development of intracranial hemorrhage. He was scheduled to undergo stereotactic radiosurgery for his metastatic brain lesions. Before this treatment could be undertaken, he became symptomatic from an intraparenchymal hemorrhage of a metastatic lesion, requiring emergent hospitalization. He had prepared an advance directive and designated a health care surrogate in anticipation of further neurologic decline. His advance directive explicitly stated that he did not wish to receive chemotherapy or radiation therapy unless there was significant medical probability of improvement. He articulated similar wishes to his niece, who was his health care surrogate.

He was estranged from the remainder of his family. His brothers had not been involved with the preparation of his advance directive or his end-of-life care discussions with his niece. When he was hospitalized with an intracranial hemorrhage, one of his brothers arrived at the hospital and reunited with the patient. The brother initially requested a plan of care that diverged from the patient's previously communicated wishes, asking the patient to receive whole-brain radiation.

Deterioration in the patient's neurological condition with development of expressive aphasia and disorientation made it difficult to discuss treatment options in detail. However, when asked about whole-brain radiation therapy, the patient consistently declined treatment. This request was in line with his statement regarding chemotherapy and radiation therapy in his advance directive and in his prior conversations with his niece. Nevertheless, his brother requested radiation therapy to be administered while the patient continued to decline treatment.

A psychiatry evaluation helped elucidate that the patient understood the proposed treatment plan along with the consequences of refusing treatment, despite his language deficit. He was able to articulate that he did not want to receive radiation and that refusing treatment may hasten his death. It was ultimately concluded that he had capacity to decline radiation therapy. His brother's inclusion during the psychiatry evaluation ensured that family members were part of the discussion and that they understood the patient's goals of care.

His prior statements in his advance directive and his conversations with his niece were consistent with his refusal of radiation therapy, which may have obviated the need for a capacity evaluation. However, involvement of the psychiatry team both gave the patient a chance to request a different plan of care and allowed the entire family to understand the treatment plan. Ultimately, he was transitioned to hospice and died several days later, having reunited with his brother and accompanied by his niece. Preparation of an advance directive and having thorough end-of-life discussions with his health care surrogate helped him receive care that was in accordance with his wishes.

Suggested Reading

1. Gillick MR. Advance care planning. *N Engl J Med.* 2004 Jan 1;**350**(1):7–8.

2. Quill TE, Abernethy AP. Generalist plus specialist palliative care – creating a sustainable model. *NENgl J Med.* 2013 Mar 28;**368**(13):1173–5.

3. Norden AD, Wen PY, Kesari S. Brain metastases. *Curr Opin Neurol.* 2005;**18**(6):654–61.

4. Owonikoko TK, Arbiser J, Zelnak A, Shu HK, Robin AM, Kalkanis SN, Whitsett TG, Salhia B, Tran NL, Ryken T, Moore MK, Egan KM, Olson JJ. Current approaches to the treatment of metastatic brain tumours. *Nature Reviews Clinical Oncology.* 2014;**11**: 203–22.

5. Davies MA, Lui P, McIntyre S, Kim KB, Papadopoulos N, Hwu WJ, Hwu P, Bedikian A. Prognostic factors for survival in melanoma patients with brain metastases. *Cancer.* 2010;**117**(8):1687–96.

6. Mandybur TI. Intracranial hemorrhage caused by metastatic tumors. *Neurology.* 1977;**27**(7):650.

7. Taillibert S, Delattre JY. Palliative care in patients with brain metastases. *Curr Opin Oncol.* 2005;**17**(6):588–92.

Taking Flight at the End of Life

Jessica Besbris

Clinical History

A 65-year-old woman with a one-year history of multifocal primary CNS lymphoma presented to the hospital with acute altered mental status and severe low back pain. She had already progressed through first- and second-line agents and she was on her third course of chemotherapy; since diagnosis she had been maintained on steroids for reduction of intracranial pressure. Her last cycle of chemotherapy was postponed due to leukopenia. Several days before she was to resume therapy, she developed confusion and lethargy, and her family brought her to the emergency room for evaluation. An MRI brain was obtained and it revealed a marked increase in the size and number of her lesions, with associated edema and midline shift. She also mentioned recent onset of severe low back pain, and MRI of the T/L spine revealed multilevel acute compression fractures that did not appear to be infiltrated by tumor. Despite having had progressive gait instability over the past year (requiring use of a wheelchair most of the time), there was no recent fall history, and the fractures were assumed to be related to long-standing steroid use, which could not be tapered due to the presence of cerebral edema.

Examination

She was afebrile with normal vital signs. She had a cushingoid appearance. She was somnolent but arousable, oriented x4, and able to follow commands. Her pupils were equal, round, and reactive to light, but she had bilateral ptosis to mid-pupil. She had full range of extraocular movements and her cranial nerve exam was otherwise unremarkable. Strength was 4+/5 throughout, with the exception of her proximal right upper extremity and bilateral proximal lower extremities, which had 4−/5 strength. Sensation to pinprick was mildly reduced in the right lower extremity, but there was no sensory level. She had mild dysmetria on right heel to shin testing. Her gait examination was initially deferred due to severe back pain with movement. She did not have spinous process tenderness but was very tender to palpation in her paraspinous muscles bilaterally, and these muscles were noted to be in spasm from T10 to L2.

Palliative Domain of Care

Physical Aspects of Care – Pain

She had substantial pain from her multilevel compression fractures. Her pain was exacerbated by movement and by prolonged sitting. She noted mild relief with acetaminophen 1,000 mg that she had been using at home. It was clear from her examination that paraspinal muscle spasm was a major component of her pain, perhaps more so than the bony pain itself. She denied anxiety or depression, which might contribute to total pain. In fact, she endorsed being at peace with her illness. She was a Jehovah's Witness and she explained that her faith allowed her to reach a point of acceptance because "this is all temporary, and we will all be together in paradise."

Palliative Care Discussion

Given her extensive intracranial edema and altered mentation, she received a loading dose of dexamethasone 10 mg IV x1, and her baseline steroid dosing was increased to 6 mg IV twice per day. Her mentation improved and she was more able to participate in medical decision-making. She and her family were told of her poor prognosis, and they were informed that fourth-line chemotherapy was unlikely to result in significant improvement and that it may result in substantial side effects. She stated that she did not wish to pursue further chemotherapy, hoping to return to her home (a one-and-a-half-hour flight away) to initiate hospice. Her neuro-oncologist estimated that she would likely live only a few more weeks. She hoped to leave the hospital as soon as possible so that she could catch her return flight and spend as much time as possible in the comfort of her home.

The biggest barrier to discharge and travel was pain control. She was described by family as "stoic" and she did admit that she often minimized her pain because she did not wish to take a lot of medications. However, her trip home would involve multiple transfers between wheelchairs and airplane seats, as well as prolonged sitting, both of which were expected to exacerbate her pain and make the trip quite difficult. She acknowledged that some degree of pain medication would be needed in order for her to tolerate the journey. She was hesitant to use opiate medications as she feared being overly sedated during travel, and she also had a questionable history of opioid allergy (rash with oxycodone and hydrocodone). She also did not wish to undergo any invasive procedures.

Hospital Course

On hospital day two, she was started on acetaminophen 1,000 mg by mouth three times per day, lidocaine patches (12 hours on and 12 hours off), menthol-containing ointment three times per day during the time the lidocaine patch was off, and heating pads to be used on an as-needed basis. She was given a "test dose" of hydromorphone 1 mg by mouth to assess for drug allergy while she was in the safe environment of the hospital. Occupational therapy was consulted to assess her ability to travel, and to teach her and her family compensatory techniques to ease her pain during the trip.

On hospital day three, she reported that her pain was moderately improved, however when practicing transfers and prolonged sitting with occupational therapy in preparation for her flight, she noted severe pain that persisted until she returned to bed. Given the absence of an allergic reaction to hydromorphone, she was started on hydromorphone 2 mg by mouth every four hours as needed and cyclobenzaprine 5 mg by mouth three times per day as needed, with instructions to take the two in combination 15–30 minutes prior to her next session with occupational therapy.

On hospital day four, she reported that with use of the aforementioned regimen she was able to transfer to her wheelchair and remain upright for three hours. She was not pain-free during this time, but she reported the pain was tolerable and her cognition was not clouded. She was able to enjoy lunch in the hospital plaza with her family, and she left the next morning for the airport. Her family called the following evening to report that she had tolerated travel well and she was met at her home by the hospice agency that had been contacted prior to her discharge.

General Remarks

In addressing this patient's pain control, it was necessary to consider multiple factors in accordance with her goals of care. The regimen chosen had to be quickly and safely titrated within just a few days to allow sufficient pain control for travel. She preferred to use non-opioid analgesics as much as possible, to minimize the dosage of opiates required. Any drugs with the potential to be sedating were started at the lowest doses possible, and multiple topical treatments were utilized to minimize systemic side effects. Opioid allergy also had to be ruled out. While kyphoplasty can be used to treat pain resulting from compression fractures, she did not wish to pursue invasive procedures. Occupational therapy was utilized to ensure that she could travel safely and to teach her non-pharmacologic strategies to ease pain during transfers. Finally, a careful examination revealed that her primary pain generator was her paraspinal muscle spasm, rather than bony pain, allowing a targeted treatment approach with muscle relaxants.

Suggested Reading

1. Cohen SP, Argoff CE, Carragee EJ. Management of low back pain. *BMJ*. 2009;**338**:100–6.

2. Gordon DB, Dahl JL, Miaskowski C. American Pain Society recommendations for improving the quality of acute and cancer pain management. *Arch Intern Med*. 2005;**165**(14):1574–80.

Palliative care for infants and children with serious or life-threatening neurological illnesses involves managing symptoms, supporting family members, improving care coordination, and providing assistance with decision-making in the setting of prognostic uncertainty [1, 2]. The palliative care interdisciplinary team engages with the child and with the entire family, as the care unit may include multiple people such as parents, siblings, grandparents, and other family members [2]. Common referrals to palliative care involve children who have genetic, congenital, or neuromuscular diseases [3]. The complexity of the condition, prognosis, and the trajectory of the disease are also considered at the time of consultation [2].

Discussions with the family and medical teams regarding prognosis, the risks and benefits of life-prolonging care, advance care planning, and hospice care in pediatric patients can be challenging. Palliative care teams can assist with eliciting the child and family's understanding of the illness, identifying their goals for their medical care, and aligning the available treatment options with their goals [2, 4]. Assisting with conflict resolution, between family members or family and care teams, is another role of the palliative team [4]. As in the adult population, palliative care integration is recommended at the time of diagnosis, when the disease progresses, or when refractory symptoms develop [2, 4].

Palliative Concepts at the Time of Diagnosis: Disease-Specific Considerations

- Pediatric neurology

  - Advance directives

  - Tracheostomy/PEG/Ventriculoperitoneal shunt
  - Accommodations for mobility impairment or cognitive dysfunction
  - Symptom management
  - Effect of the disease on siblings/parents/other family
  - Child life specialist integration
  - General considerations:

    · Discussion regarding the disease
    · Symptom management
    · Mood and coping
    · Progression of disease/disease trajectory
    · Advance care planning

Suggested Reading

1. Lemmon ME, Bidegain M, Boss RD. Palliative care in neonatal neurology: Robust support for infants, families and clinicians. *Journal of Perinatology: Official Journal of the California Perinatal Association.* 2016;**36**(5):331–7.

2. Moore D, Sheetz J. Pediatric palliative care consultation. *Pediatric Clinics of North America.* 2014;**61**(4):735–47.

3. Feudtner C, Kang TI, Hexem KR, et al. Pediatric palliative care patients: A prospective multicenter cohort study. *Pediatrics.* 2011;**127**(6):1094–1101.

4. Boss R, Nelson J, Weissman D, et al. Integrating palliative care into the PICU: A report from the Improving Palliative Care in the ICU Advisory Board. *Pediatric Critical Care Medicine: A Journal of the Society of Critical Care Medicine and the World Federation of Pediatric Intensive and Critical Care Societies.* 2014;**15**(8):762–7.

Chapter 42

Not Another Shunt Revision

Alva Roche-Green

Clinical History

CC is an eight-year-old girl with a history of congenital hydrocephalus diagnosed in the newborn nursery after recognition of an enlarged head circumference followed by confirmatory imaging consistent with communicating hydrocephalus. At that time, due to the working diagnosis of communicating hydrocephalus, there was no need for placement of a ventriculoperitoneal (VP) shunt, but plans for close neurosurgical follow-up were made in case future interventions were needed. Unfortunately, her mother failed to follow up as scheduled and she did not present again for medical attention until after her first birthday. At that time she was noted to have marked malnutrition and global developmental delay with marked craniomegaly and a "heart-shaped skull" due to worsening hydrocephalus. She was hospitalized for further intervention, including placement of a VP shunt and a feeding tube. A CT of the brain showed bilateral massive enlargement of the lateral ventricles, splaying of sutures, and marked cortical thinning.

Despite these interventions she had no neurologic improvement and she was classified as having severe neurologic impairment of static nature with evidence of cerebral palsy. Because of medical neglect on the part of her birth mother, she was placed in foster care and eventually adopted by a family who was able to take care of her significant medical needs. She received aggressive rehabilitative services.

Examination

She was awake and smiling. There was macrocephaly with frontal bossing and scalp veins were prominent. Her tone was increased in all extremities.

Palliative Domains of Care

Ethical and Legal Aspects of Care: Decision-making at the end of life in children

"End-of-life care for children is not ethically straightforward and the ethical challenges it poses for society and for health care professionals are complex and difficult. Children are not small adults and should not be treated as such" [2]. As a result, the adaptation of adult ethical principles for medical decision-making to deal with the special circumstance of dealing with children/adolescents at the end-of-life has been challenging. For example, when we discuss goals of care or end-of-life decisions, autonomy is the central ethical principle used in caring for adults. This requires informed consent or at least "informed assent" of the patient. However in pediatric care, given the varying ages and developmental stages of chronically ill children, this is not always feasible. It is impossible, for example, to understand the goals, values, and beliefs of a child who has not developed those characteristics due to young age or developmental delay. This requires the surrogate decision maker with no advanced directive or guidance from the child to make decisions in the child's best interest, or to rely on the ethical principles of beneficence and non-maleficence. These decisions are often made via a shared decision-making process involving the family and the medical team.

CCs parents were faced with a procedure that had the potential to cause their daughter pain without the potential to improve her quality. After thoroughly discussing all of the treatment options available with CC's medical team, they made the choice not to have her VP shunt revised/replaced. This decision was made in what they felt was her best interest. CC's family opted to focus on her quality of life and to pursue comfort. This was a decision supported by CC's care team, including her palliative medicine team who continued to care for her, and they provided the best quality of life possible until her death.

Structure and Process of Care: Pediatric Palliative Care and Hospice

Pediatric palliative care is an approach to care for infants, children, and adolescents suffering from chronic and life-limiting medical conditions. The focus is to improve the quality of life for those patients and their families. Hospice care is an extension of those services with a greater focus on end-of-life care. Approximately 53,000 children die each year in the United States and at least 400,000 more live every day with chronic, life-threatening conditions. Despite the growth of pediatric hospice and palliative care services, pediatric patients make up less than 1 percent of patients served by hospice programs each year (Figure 42.1).

Data published in 2015 based on a 2007 survey of children's hospitals revealed that across the United States, 69 percent of children's hospitals reported having a palliative medicine team and 30 percent of those programs also offered home visit services. Many hospice programs are also serving younger patients. Data from the National Hospice and Palliative Care Organization's 2015 report reveals that 78 percent of hospices report serving pediatric patients with more than 35 percent having specific pediatric programs in place. For those hospices without a dedicated pediatric team, 21.7 percent have a specialist providing only pediatric services. Additionally, 14.1 percent of hospices report that they provide pediatric palliative care services.

Palliative Care Discussion

The palliative team visited CC at her family's home. CC was sitting in her usual chair, which is a toddler car seat. She appeared comfortable with no seizure activity noted. Vitals signs were within normal limits. Her eyes were closed and she did not respond to verbal or tactile stimuli, which her mother notes she did previously. No cough or respiratory distress or secretions. A left-sided VP shunt was noted with no

obvious fractures on palpation. Attempts to compress the shunt valve were met with significant resistance and shunt dysfunction was suspected. Her antiepileptic medications were increased and she was evaluated by her neurosurgeon with imaging.

Shunt malfunction was confirmed and other etiologies of the decline in her mental status such as infection were ruled out. A VP shunt revision was recommended. Her mother reports that CC's shunt had been replaced three times previously, with the last revision about five years ago. Each shunt revision was associated with pain and discomfort during recovery as well as a decline in CC's level of interaction. Her mom was concerned about putting CC through another procedure that would keep her alive but that would be unlikely to improve her quality of life.

After extensive discussions within CC's family and with her neurologist, neurosurgeon, and pediatric palliative care specialist, the decision was made not to replace CC's shunt and to focus on her comfort with a prognosis of a few weeks to a few months. CC passed away peacefully at home with her family three months later.

Clinical Course

At baseline she was nonverbal, non-ambulatory, and required total care. Despite her limitations, her family reported that she was a happy child who was able to laugh, smile, and interact with her family in a meaningful way. She was able to have some oral intake for pleasure, but she continued to require enteral feeds to maintain adequate nutrition. She was enrolled in pediatric palliative care services due to her complex medical needs and for the emotional

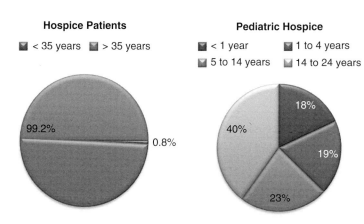

Figure 42.1 Stratification of hospice patients by age Adapted from the National Hospice and Palliative Medicine Organizations "Facts & Figures on Pediatric Palliative Care and Hospice." 2015

support needed by her adoptive family, who provided all appropriate medical care.

Just prior to her sixth birthday, her family noted that she became less interactive and she began to have a marked decrease in oral intake. Her symptoms coincided with an upper respiratory tract infection, which for her usually resulted in similar symptoms. However as the respiratory symptoms resolved over several weeks her neurological status continued to decline to the point where she was minimally responsive and had no oral intake. A palliative care home visit was requested.

General Remarks

Early involvement of palliative care services in the care of children with chronic medical conditions is recommended. This is especially true for those with serious neurologic impairment due to structural or chromosomal abnormalities, congenital syndromes, inborn errors of metabolism, and acute neurologic injury. The prognoses of these patients varies based on the age of onset and severity of symptoms, but each of these patients and their families face a lifetime of complex care that can have both a physical and a psychological impact on the family. While medical care has improved the quality of life of thousands of children and adolescents with severe neurological impairment, treatment options can also be burdensome and in some situations without measurable benefit. The interdisciplinary approach to palliative care can be essential to supporting patients and families as they learn to cope with the emotional high and lows, the hope and despair. Palliative care supports patients and families along the entire continuum of chronic disease by promoting the best quality of life that can be obtained while also being there to support the tough decisions at the end of life and beyond with bereavement support.

Suggested Reading

1. National Hospice and Palliative Medicine Organizations. "Facts & Figures on Pediatric Palliative Care and Hospice." 2015. www.nhpco.org/sites/default/files/public/quality/Pediatric_Facts-Figures.pdf.

2. Doka KJ, Tucci AS. *Living with Grief: Children and Adolescents*. Washington, DC: Hospice Foundation of America; 2008.

3. Hauer, JM. *Caring for Children Who Have Severe Neurological Impairment: A Life with Grace*. Baltimore: Johns Hopkins University Press, 2013.

4. Parker, DC, Protus, BM, O'Neill Hunt, M, Penfield Winters, J. *Pediatric Palliative Care Consultation: Guidelines for Effective Management of Symptoms*. Montgomery, AL: HospiScript Services, 2014.

Intrathecal Baclofen for Severe Spasticity

Shayna Rich and Maisha T. Robinson

Clinical History

An 18-year-old man had presented to an emergency department eight years earlier with diplopia and "a funny sensation" on the right side of his body. His evaluation included an MRI brain, which revealed a cavernous malformation in the left midbrain (Figure 43.1). He was given an infusion of high-dose steroids and his symptoms resolved the following day.

He subsequently had approximately yearly episodes of severe headache, diplopia, and numbness of the right side that were attributed to minor acute hemorrhages. His symptoms remained responsive to steroids with a return to baseline within a few days. He continued to have yearly clinic follow-up and serial MRIs for surveillance with no significant changes. He had episodes of poorly controlled anger related to frustration with his diagnosis, and he had a history of opioid abuse.

At 17 years old, he presented to an emergency department due to headaches, diplopia, and right hemisensory loss, secondary to an acute brainstem hemorrhage related to his cavernoma. He was treated with a conservative approach with high-dose steroids and he had a full recovery. Following extensive counseling regarding his options, he underwent elective surgical excision of the vascular malformation (Figures 43.2 and 43.3).

In the immediate postoperative period, he was more somnolent than anticipated, and several days after the procedure, he was noted to have fixed and dilated pupils. He had a slow but steady improvement in his cognitive status until he was following commands. However, on postoperative day five, he began developing declining mental status and hypertonia. The hypertonia began on his right side and progressed to the left side. This gradually worsened over the course of months.

He was medically stabilized and discharged to a pediatric rehabilitation center. Unfortunately, his potential for rehabilitation was limited and his motor function continued to worsen. He was only able to elevate his left eyebrow, smile on the left side, and extend his tongue. Baclofen was initiated and

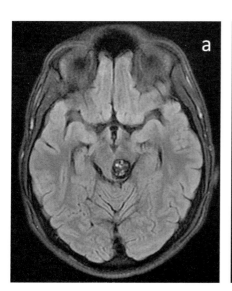
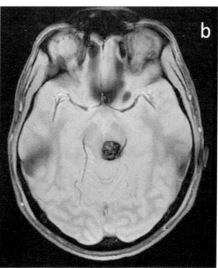

Figure 43.1 MRI brain (a) fluid attenuation inversion recovery; (b) gradient echo revealing a left dorsal midbrain cavernoma

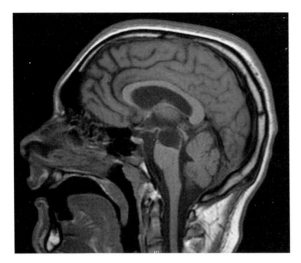

Figure 43.2 MRI brain (Sagittal T1) showing the postoperative resection cavity in the midbrain

titrated up to 20 mg three times a day, but he continued to have severe generalized spasticity.

He presented to the outpatient clinic for a second opinion and he was subsequently admitted to the hospital. The neurologist discussed with him and with his family that it was highly unlikely that his neurologic outcome could be significantly improved with surgical intervention. However, his treatment plan would focus on speech augmentation, occupational and physical therapy, and management of his spasticity and pain.

Examination

He was alert and sitting in a wheelchair in a decorticate posture. He was able to follow commands to stick out his tongue, smile, and raise his eyebrow. His pupils were fixed and dilated, but he blinked to threat bilaterally. He had right hemiplegia, and left hemiparesis with minimal movement in his left hand and thumb. He was unable to move his eyes at all. He had right hemisensory loss, and brisk reflexes on the left.

Palliative Domain of Care

Physical Aspects of Care – Management of spasticity

He had no ability to recover neurologically, given the irreversible damage to the brainstem. Efforts were focused on optimizing quality of life and maximizing function. Primary concerns included his prominent symptoms of pain and spasticity. He also had frequent

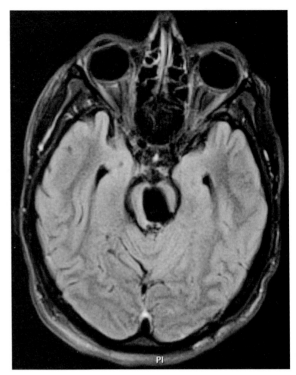

Figure 43.3 MRI brain (axial fluid attenuated inversion recovery) showing the postoperative resection cavity in the midbrain

episodes of overwhelming diaphoresis, tachypnea, tachycardia, and dystonia. These episodes were diagnosed as paroxysmal autonomic instability with dystonia (PAID), which was subsequently controlled with scheduled clonidine. The palliative care team was consulted to discuss goals of care and to improve his symptom control.

Palliative Care Discussion

An effort was made to include him as much as possible in discussions, although this was limited based on the difficulties with communication. Most information was provided by his mother. She stated that they had understood that he had chosen the surgery to avoid a catastrophic bleed, but that he had permanent neurologic impairment as a result of the high-risk surgery. They hoped to reverse his paralysis, but they knew that this was unlikely. On questioning, he blinked to indicate that "this is hell" and he acknowledged that he was in pain. His pain was related to his spasticity, which was suboptimally controlled. His baclofen had helped in a minor way with his spasticity, but his spasticity remained a major limitation of his ability to be manipulated and to participate in physical therapy. He and his mother were willing to change medications or to adjust them in an attempt to improve his functioning.

Treatment Course

Neurosurgery and the pain teams were consulted for the consideration of an intrathecal baclofen pump. He underwent a test dose of intrathecal baclofen with 50 mcg. He had an evaluation by physical therapy before and after the test dose. The intrathecal dose yielded a drastic reduction in his baseline dystonia, and it improved his ability to relax and to allow for passive range of motion.

An adjustable intrathecal pump containing baclofen was implanted and set for an initial dose with 50 mcg/day. Over the following days of hospitalization, the pump was gradually increased to 90 mcg/day. With the improvement in tone, he was better able to participate in therapy. He was discharged to inpatient rehabilitation to continue with physical, occupational, and speech therapy.

General Remarks

Spinal drug delivery allows direct delivery into the epidural or intrathecal space where it can have a direct effect on the dorsal horn. Given the relative lack of dispersal, there is a much lower serum blood level of the drug and it permits a much lower dose of the drug to be used for a similar effect. Because the serum blood level is the main determinant of systemic side effects, intrathecal drug delivery allows an effective dose of the drug to be given while minimizing intolerable side effects. It is helpful for patients with generalized symptoms as this method cannot localize medication delivery.

Options for spinal drug delivery include epidural or intrathecal routes. The epidural route is best used for short-term drug delivery, as it has a higher rate of long-term complications. Intrathecal drug delivery allows for a lower dose of medication (one-tenth of that used in epidural delivery), as it can provide the drug directly to the dorsal horn. With the lower dose, there is less risk of side effects and less need for refilling of medications. It is also less affected by the presence of epidural metastatic disease or other epidural pathology.

Absolute contraindications for placement of a spinal catheter for drug delivery include coagulopathy, sepsis, or infection near the catheter site. Complications include headaches, adverse reactions to the medications, or those related to hardware placement, including catheter kinking, disconnections, dislodgement, or infection.

Patients who have chronic symptoms may benefit from placement of a long-term method of drug delivery with a pump placed internally. Patients should be considered for intrathecal pump placement only if they have a life expectancy of several months or more, and a good performance status. Patients should be evaluated prior to pump placement to ensure that they have realistic goals and that they will be compliant with follow-up visits for routine pump refills. Patients should not be approved for pump placement if they have concerns related to paying for medical costs, unmanaged mental health problems, or a history of noncompliance.

Spinal drug delivery is used as an option for treatment of muscle spasticity with baclofen, or for pain management with medications, including fentanyl, morphine, or hydromorphone. Determining whether a spinal drug delivery system is appropriate is based on clinical considerations, but the decision of specific systems depends on the available expertise, volume of implant needed (based on daily dose and drug concentration), logistics, and payer approval.

Intrathecal Baclofen

Intrathecal baclofen is indicated when chronic muscle spasticity interferes with comfort, function, activities of daily living, mobility, positioning, or caregiver assistance. Common diagnoses for patients who may benefit from this mode of medication delivery include severe head injury or spinal cord trauma, multiple sclerosis, cerebral palsy, or spinal spondylosis. It need not be reserved for patients who fail other approaches, as it may provide a more-targeted intervention and decrease the dose of medication needed.

Patients under consideration for intrathecal baclofen pumps should be given a test dose with a 50-mcg bolus provided by a removable intrathecal catheter (or 25 mcg in very small children). The patient's spasticity should be measured prior to the test dose, and then at least twice within four hours after the dose is given. Patients should also have cardiopulmonary parameters monitored frequently during the first two hours post-injection, to ensure that they are stable. Observation should continue until the patient is stable and returns to baseline. If patients do not have a measurable response to the 50 mcg dose, then a dose of 75 or 100 mcg should be tried 24 hours later.

Following a successful trial, patients can have an intrathecal pump implanted, usually with the reservoir placed under the skin of the abdomen. The initial daily dose is usually planned to be twice that of the effective screening dose, unless the response to the screening dose was long-lasting (> eight hours), then it can be used as the daily dose. Inpatients can have the dose adjusted by 10–30 percent daily if the cause of spasticity is of spinal origin and if the patient is an adult, but it should be limited to 5–15 percent daily if the cause is of cerebral origin or if the patient is a child. Outpatients who will have less frequent adjustment can have step increases. Assessment of the response to the dose change should be performed within 24 hours.

For many patients, the goal of placing a baclofen pump is to eliminate oral antispasmodics. These patients can have their antispasmodics weaned prior to the trial or following the pump placement. These medications should be weaned individually over time. Oral baclofen should be the first antispasmodic weaned, to limit the risk of adverse effects while the pump is being titrated.

Suggested Reading

1. Boster AL, Bennett SE, Bilsky GS, et al. Best practices for intrathecal baclofen therapy: Screening test. *Neuromodulation*. 2016 Aug;**19**(6):623–31.

2. Pope JE, Deer TR, Bruel BM, Falowski S. Clinical uses of intrathecal therapy and its placement in the pain care algorithm. *Practical Pain Management*. 2016 Feb 23.

3. Reisfield GM, Wilson GR; National Residency End-of-Life Curriculum Project. Intrathecal drug therapy for pain #98. *Journal of Palliative Medicine*. 2004 Feb;**7**(1):76.

4. Saulino M, Ivanhoe CB, McGuire JR, et al. Best practices for intrathecal baclofen therapy: Patient selection. *Neuromodulation*. 2016 Aug;**19**(6):607–15.

Multiple sclerosis is a chronic disease that leads to progressive disability, and palliative care has been suggested as an approach to manage symptoms and improve quality of life [1]. A variety of physical and psychological symptoms can impact patients' lives, such as fatigue, mobility issues, pain, drowsiness, and depression [1–3]. Broader issues involving structuring the day, new life roles, progression of disease, and advance care planning also need to be addressed, as patients desire to discuss end-of-life issues with their providers [4, 5].

Palliative care can be integrated into the care for patients with multiple sclerosis at the time of diagnosis, and triggers for more advanced palliative care consultation may be symptom-related or disease-stage-related [1]. The ideal timing of when to initiate a consultation has not been established, but more formal assessments may be appropriate when significant changes in function occur, such as when a patient requires nursing support, when the symptom burden is significant, or when changes in prognosis are discussed [1]. Psychological assessments in patients with multiple sclerosis are necessary given the high rate of mood disorders and risk of suicide in this population [2]. Identifying social supports and positive coping strategies may reduce the risk of depression [2].

Uncertainty exists regarding the role of palliative care in the management of patients with multiple sclerosis [5]. Increasing awareness of the breadth and depth of palliative care resources among multiple sclerosis patients and providers may improve access to – and utilization of – these services [1, 5].

Palliative Concepts at the Time of Diagnosis: Disease-Specific Considerations

- Multiple sclerosis
  - Advance directives

- Accommodations for mobility impairment or cognitive dysfunction
- Symptom management
- Social support
- Caregiver support
- General considerations:
  - Discussion regarding the disease
  - Symptom management
  - Mood and coping
  - Progression of disease/disease trajectory
  - Advance care planning

Suggested Reading

1. Strupp J, Romotzky V, Galushko M, Golla H, Voltz R. Palliative care for severely affected patients with multiple sclerosis: When and why? Results of a Delphi survey of health care professionals. *Journal of Palliative Medicine*. 2014;**17**(10):1128–36.

2. Siegert RJ, Abernethy DA. Depression in multiple sclerosis: A review. *Journal of Neurology, Neurosurgery, and Psychiatry*. 2005;**76**(4):469–75.

3. Higginson IJ, Hart S, Silber E, Burman R, Edmonds P. Symptom prevalence and severity in people severely affected by multiple sclerosis. *Journal of Palliative Care*. 2006;**22**(3): 158–65.

4. Strupp J, Voltz R, Golla H. Opening locked doors: Integrating a palliative care approach into the management of patients with severe multiple sclerosis. *Multiple Sclerosis (Houndmills, Basingstoke, England)*. 2016;**22**(1):13–18.

5. Golla H, Galushko M, Pfaff H, Voltz R. Multiple sclerosis and palliative care – perceptions of severely affected multiple sclerosis patients and their health professionals: A qualitative study. *BMC Palliative Care*. 2014;**13**(1):11.

Palliative Care in Multiple Sclerosis
Navigating Chronic Disease Can Be a Difficult Pill to Swallow at a Young Age

Ludo J. Vanopdenbosch and David J. Oliver

Clinical History

A colorfully tattooed decorator was diagnosed with multiple sclerosis at age 19. The diagnosis was only made after several relapses and increasing disability. He had not sought neurological evaluation but he had tried homeopathy and exercise. An MRI scan of his brain showed multiple contrast-enhancing lesions. His clinical course, age, sex, and scan classified him as having a poor prognosis warranting aggressive therapy. He was included in a double blind, double dummy phase III clinical trial with ocrelizumab versus high dose interferon beta1a.

Examination

On presentation he was wheelchair bound, incontinent of urine, impotent, and he had diplopia. The Expanded Disability Scale Score (EDSS) which indicates increasing disability from 0 (no signs or symptoms) to 10 (death) was 6.0.

In the following year he did not experience further relapses and he recovered slowly to an EDSS of 2.5, allowing him to resume work. At 15 months into the trial, he opted out saying he did not want these medicines anymore, he had seen the light and he was convinced that the white spots on the scans would disappear with a diet based on oats. He was followed up according to the study protocol however, but without study medication.

One year later, at age 21, he experienced a severe relapse with left hemisensory loss and severe coordination problems, and on MRI there were several new lesions. He was started on natalizumab, after extensive discussion and education, with good effect, only to drop out 6 months later after an internet search had informed him of the evils of the medical industry.

Domains of Palliative Care

Ethical and Legal Aspects of Care – Poor patient compliance
Psychological Aspects of Care – Depression

An ethical question was raised: should the behavior of the patient influence treatment decisions? MS treatments are very expensive and poor adherence to treatment will make them less efficacious which could mean waste and unfair use of resources (justice). However the indication for a treatment should be based on best medical knowledge, uninfluenced by subjective elements (beneficence). Psychological problems interfering with therapy should be addressed accordingly, such as by referring the patient for psychiatric evaluation or psychotherapy. However reliability can be a factor which has to be taken into account when choosing a dangerous therapy with a risk management plan with frequent follow ups and blood analyses for several years.

Palliative Care Discussion

After a lengthy discussion, we agreed to follow him without treatment, with routine examinations and MRI scans. Initially, he was reliable, but then he disappeared for eight months. He resurfaced in the emergency room, unconscious, after being found by his father. Later he told us that he had taken 140 tablets of zopiclone that he bought over the Internet in a suicide attempt. He stayed in the intensive care unit for three days and he survived without harm.

This incident prompted a "serious talk" with the neurologist and a palliative care physician. We explored aspects of symptom control, existential issues, and social issues, about both the present situation and the foreseeable future. Chronic generalized pain due to mild spasticity was treated with low-dose baclofen. Delving into his quality of life and his mood led to a conversation about his concern regarding a lack of prospects with which to start a family. We referred him to a urologist for erectile dysfunction and to a psychiatrist for severe depression, both of whom chose non-pharmacological approaches with psychotherapy and relational therapy.

General Remarks

Palliative care is not limited to end-of-life care or to symptom control solely in the dying phase. Palliative care focuses on improving quality of life, which includes symptom management, advance care planning, care for the caregivers, and assistance with social, psychological, and existential issues, at every stage of a chronic or serious disease. Breaking points and crisis moments should trigger a reflex to have a deeper discussion with the patient and family, and to go beyond the usual consultation etiquette, which often includes asking how things are going, performing a standard neurological examination, and writing prescriptions. Palliative care principles emphasize the importance of caring for the "whole person," which often involves taking the time to explore one's future plans, wishes, sexuality, beliefs, hopes, and fears. Based on the initial or subsequent evaluations, some patients will benefit from having a specialist palliative care consultation or consultations with other specialists, such as psychiatrists. This collaborative approach to caring for a patient is often not only beneficial for the patient, but also for the teams involved.

Suicides and requests for hastened death are common in multiple sclerosis, with a hazard ratio for suicide estimated to be four times greater than in the general population. Many MS specialists have experienced unexpected suicides and unexplained traffic accidents among their patients. Addressing issues of depression, anxiety, coping, or other mood disorders is a necessary component of the management plan in this patient population. Careful attention should be given to prescribing newer antidepressants for this population with a known risk of activation and suicide, particularly in young adults.

At the present time, our decorator is in his early thirties. He is working full time and he is leading a quiet life. He has not found a long-term partner or started a family yet. He is engaged in volunteer work for the MS patient organization with yearly biking trips. He has not experienced relapses in the past two years, his brain MRI is stable, and he is not taking disease-modifying drugs. However, he is monitored closely because the risk for relapse or MRI disease activity is high, at which stage we will probably propose to him a novel treatment with ocrelizumab IV twice a year.

Suggested Reading

1. Pompili M, Forte A, Palermo M. Suicide risk in multiple sclerosis: A systematic review of current literature. *Journal of Psychosomatic Research*. 2012;**73**:, 411–17.

2. Siegert R, Abernethy D. Depression in multiple sclerosis: A review. *J Neurol Neurosurg Psychiatry*. 2005;**76**(4):469–75.

3. Depression: National Multiple Sclerosis Society. Available open access online: www.nationalmssociety.org/Symptoms-Diagnosis/MS-Symptoms/Depression. Accessed July 10, 2017.

45

The Perils of Late Advance Care Planning in Multiple Sclerosis

Ludo J. Vanopdenbosch and David J. Oliver

Clinical History

Ingrid is a 69-year-old woman with multiple sclerosis (MS). She was diagnosed decades ago and she was treated with all available disease-modifying drugs as they became available throughout the years, including mitoxantrone and natalizumab. She had worked as a secretary in a general practitioner's (GP) office in her twenties but she was forced to stop due to increasing disability. Years ago she entered the secondary progressive stage and she is now wheelchair bound with an Expanded Disability Scale Score of 7.0, indicating moderate disability. Disease-modifying drugs were stopped several years ago. She is now taking oxycodone for pain, baclofen for spasticity, anticholinergics for stress incontinence, metformin for type 2 diabetes, beta-blockers for hypertension, a sleeping pill, and estrogen replacement. She presents for evaluation because she has noticed that very slowly she is losing strength in her arms and transfers from the wheelchair to a seat or to the toilet are becoming more and more difficult. She is convinced that she cannot live in her house with her partner, who is still working, when she cannot transfer independently. She also states that she has increasing memory concerns with annoying forgetfulness.

Examination

She is an obese woman who appears well groomed. She is sitting in an electric wheelchair. She is awake and alert, oriented to time and place. Her primary gaze is divergent; visual fields are full to confrontation. Her speech is dysarthric but intelligible. Strength is 4/5 in the upper extremities and 1/5 in the lower extremities with marked spasticity and hyperactive reflexes; Babinski's sign is present bilaterally. She has an indwelling catheter and no decubitus ulcers.

Domain of Palliative Care

Structure and Process of Care – Discussing prognosis and clarifying goals of care

Palliative Care Discussion

Her request for treatment and her fears of loss of independence triggered a deeper discussion, a "serious disease talk." We explored what she knew about the future and how multiple sclerosis will undoubtedly affect her more in the coming years. She seemed to be very realistic. She was thinking about the future and she was very scared of having to leave her home and be taken care of in residential care. We asked her permission to contact a residential care home that specialized in advanced MS so they could organize a tour of their facilities, but she declined. We offered to talk to her partner, whom we had never met despite our caring for her for years, but she again declined. Her memory problems became more obvious over the years and she refused neurocognitive testing because of a perceived lack of therapeutic possibilities. Despite this, we thought that she had the capacity to engage in advance care planning. She indicated that she desired no further hospitalizations and that she preferred to stay at home with her GP's care in the event of serious infections. She documented her preferences to not be resuscitated at the time of cardiopulmonary arrest and to not be mechanically ventilated. She expressed a sense of relief at having had this conversation.

Clinical Course

Less than a couple of weeks later, during the annual leave of her treating neurologist, she was brought to the emergency room (ER) and bilateral bacterial pneumonia, possibly due to aspiration, was diagnosed. The advance care directive was retrieved in the electronic patient files and when confronted with it, she denied ever having written it up, and she requested full therapy, including ventilation if needed. Her daughter accompanied her at the ER and she also denied ever having heard of advance care directives. The patient was put on IV antibiotics, she received a bronchoscopy to remove mucous plugs and to assess for aspirated food, and she was ventilated for two days in the intensive care unit. She made a full recovery.

We requested a palliative care team intervention to explore her wishes but also to address unmet symptoms and to assess for caregiver burden. There is evidence that such a palliative care intervention in advanced multiple sclerosis is useful. Irene Higginson has studied this in the United Kingdom and found measurable improvements in symptom control: pain, nausea, oral pain, insomnia, and significantly reducing caregiver burden. She also found this service to be cost-effective.

General Remarks

Advance care directives are legal documents that provide guidance for life-prolonging care when a person loses capacity to make medical decisions at the end of life. They have advantages but also limitations, as illustrated. Impaired communication, disagreement between doctors and caregivers, cognitive problems, and the difficulty of making decisions prior to the end of life are evident limitations. While a person possesses the capacity to make medical decisions, he can contradict or change the preferences that are documented in the advance directive. As the name suggests, these directives are written in advance of when one would need it. Therefore, a person is asked to make decisions about the care that they would want in a hypothetical situation. When a person is closer to the end of life, he may make different decisions or he may prioritize his care in a different manner than what he alluded to in a prior advance directive.

Advance care planning conversations and discussions regarding treatment preferences should ideally include all relevant stakeholders – the patient, the treating physicians, caregivers, and health care surrogates. In this case, because the patient was evaluated alone at every clinic visit over the years, it was unclear how much her family understood about her condition or about her wishes for her care. In some instances, home visits can offer an opportunity to assess a patient in his own environment and to incorporate his caregivers in the discussion regarding treatment plans. This can be particularly useful for people with cognitive decline, as in this patient's case. Working in collaboration with the patient's other providers, such as his GP or community nurse, can facilitate a unified management plan and improve the continuity of care.

Suggested Reading

1. Higginson IJ, et al., Is short-term palliative care cost-effective in multiple sclerosis? A randomized phase II trial. *Journal of Pain and Symptom Management.* 2009;**38**:816–26.

2. Gruenewald D, Brodkey M, Reitman NC, Del Bene M. Opening doors: The palliative care continuum in multiple sclerosis. *A Clinical Bulletin of the Professional Resource Centre of the National Multiple Sclerosis Society.* Available online: www.nationalmssociety.org/National MSSociety/media/MSNationalFiles/Brochures/Clinical -Bulletin-Palliative-Care-2012-Final.pdf. Accessed July 10, 2017.

3. Lawrence RE, Brauner DJ. Deciding for others: Limitations of advance directives, substituted judgement, and best interest. *AMA Journal of Ethics, Virtual Mentor.* 2009;**11**(8):571–81.

Chapter 46

Comparing and Contrasting the Approach to Advance Care Planning in Multiple Sclerosis

Gabriele C. DeLuca and Joseph J. Hutchinson

Clinical History

A 60-year-old woman with a long-standing history of secondary progressive multiple sclerosis (MS), hyperthyroidism, and depression presented to the emergency department with shortness of breath and drowsiness. Her MS history dated back more than four decades with emergence of secondary progressive disease at the age of 41 years, after which she accumulated substantial neurological disability. She required the use of a wheelchair starting at the age of 47, soon after which she became completely dependent in all of her activities of daily living. By the time of presentation, she had no purposeful movement of her limbs, severe spasticity and contractures, debilitating oscillopsia and poor visual acuity, an indwelling urinary catheter, intractable constipation requiring regular enemas, and significant cognitive decline. Recent years were marked by recurrent admissions to the hospital because of complications related to her MS, including multiple bouts of sepsis secondary to urinary tract infections, bronchopneumonia, and grade IV sacral pressure sores. She required several prolonged stays on rehabilitation wards for treatment and respite care, but she was primarily cared for by her husband at home with community support. Given her inability to maintain adequate nutrition, a percutaneous endoscopic gastrostomy (PEG) was planned in the upcoming days.

She presented to the emergency department because of shortness of breath, drowsiness, and anorexia. A week prior to presentation, she was noted to be increasingly lethargic. The morning of presentation, she started to make grunting noises and she gasped for air. All of her symptoms swiftly worsened during the course of the day, prompting a visit to the hospital that evening.

Examination

She was drowsy and made incomprehensible sounds. She appeared uncomfortable using accessory muscles of respiration. She was diaphoretic, tachypneic (21 breaths per minute), and hypoxemic (SpO_2 84 percent on room air). She was tachycardic (120 beats per minute) and had a blood pressure of 140/80 mmHg. Her temperature was 37.5°C, mucous membranes were dry with a low jugular venous pulsation (JVP), and dark urine was in her catheter bag. On auscultation of her chest, course crepitations throughout her right lung and at the left lung base were noted. Her abdomen was soft but distended. A 4 cm-deep sacral pressure sore was noted. The neurological examination was significant for a depressed level of consciousness with a Glasgow Coma Score (GCS) of 10 (baseline was 12). She inconsistently followed simple commands, but she could not communicate meaningfully. The motor examination was significant for severe contractures and disuse atrophy of both upper and lower limbs. Sensory, cerebellar/coordination, and gait examinations were deferred.

Palliative Domain of Care

Structure and Processes of Care – Interdisciplinary team assessment based on patient/family goals of care; prognosis; disposition (level of care – inpatient unit, home); referral to palliative care to guide decisions about the goals of care

She had severe end-stage secondary progressive MS with significant disability. Given her complex needs, many health care professionals from a range of disciplines were involved in her care over the years, including physicians (general practice, neurology, psychiatry, rehabilitation medicine, plastic surgery, acute medicine, and intensive care), specialist nurses (multiple sclerosis, rehabilitation, and wound care), clinical psychologists, speech and language therapists, dieticians, physiotherapists, and occupational therapists. She was evaluated by multidisciplinary teams on at least seven separate occasions. However, despite her extensive and progressive morbidity and low quality of life, at no stage was a referral to palliative care made.

Palliative Care Discussion

There had been some prior discussion about the goals of care. During her multiple admissions to the rehabilitation ward over the years, she had completed several life goals questionnaires before her cognitive dysfunction became too severe, which were appropriately considered in her package of care. On review of the medical record, the rehabilitation team had recommended full active care and treatment within the two years prior to the current admission. Although multiple health care providers were involved in her care subsequent to this, there was no further documentation about goals of care, even though her clinical condition continued to worsen. That being said, a do-not-attempt cardio-pulmonary resuscitation (DNA CPR) form was completed during an admission for bronchopneumonia the year prior and once again during the current admission after discussion by her admitting acute medical consultant with her husband and daughters.

During her last admission, the acute medicine team initially identified noninvasive ventilation for respiratory failure as the ceiling of care. Accordingly, she was admitted to the resuscitation room and her case discussed with an intensive care consultant. At that point, a discussion between the medical team and family about her baseline level of function and quality of life ensued with conflicting opinions between family members emerging. Some family members believed that she had some quality of life, thereby warranting full medical treatment, while others were less certain about this approach given her significant morbidity. After further discussion a few hours later and continued clinical decline, it was decided by the acute medicine and intensive care consultants (in consultation with the family) that noninvasive ventilation would not be in the patient's best interests. Early advance care planning with the palliative care team could have helped guide these discussions.

Clinical Course

She was admitted to the acute medicine service. A diagnosis of respiratory failure secondary to bronchopneumonia was made, prompting institution of supplemental oxygen and intravenous co-amoxicillin/clavulanic acid. Given concern of pulmonary embolism, treatment dose dalteparin was also initiated. Initially, noninvasive ventilation was deemed as the ceiling of appropriate care should her respiratory failure worsen. However, given her significant debility and worsening clinical status, this was no longer seen as appropriate after a conversation with the family a few hours later. Her family also agreed that a DNA CPR with a focus on comfort was most appropriate at this stage.

Her respiratory function continued to deteriorate rapidly over the next several hours and she suffered respiratory arrest. Scant secretions were removed by suction and high-flow oxygen was administered. Cardiac arrest ensued. She was pronounced dead. Her family agreed to donate her brain and spinal cord for research and education

General Remarks

Early palliative care input and intervention may have helped focus her goals of care and outline coordinated strategies to facilitate them. Her quality of life was very poor. She lacked capacity to make her own decisions, could not interact meaningfully with those around her, and was completely dependent on others for her basic needs. Her care was fragmented and the overall goals of care were not clearly defined. The mobilization of a palliative care approach could have helped optimize symptom management and frame realistic expectations about care needs and outcomes. This strategy would likely have preempted emergent and distressing discussions about the use of noninvasive ventilation during the acute admission and may have likely put into context the value of PEG insertion at this stage of her disease. It might have also avoided a visit to the emergency department, with care instead being focused in the community. The palliative care team could have been an effective consulting service with regard to symptom management, goals of care, caregiver support, and end-of-life care (Figure 46.1).

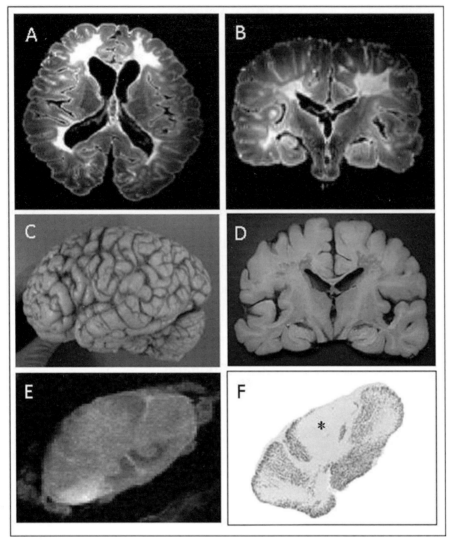

Figure 46.1 Radiographic, macroscopic, and microscopic views of the postmortem brain and spinal cord of the deceased patient featured in the case. T2-weighted MRI brain scans of the postmortem brain *ex situ* in the axial (A) and coronal (B) planes reveal extensive, confluent white matter lesions in the periventricular and juxtacortical regions along with considerable cerebral atrophy. Macroscopic view of the left lateral hemisphere (C) demonstrates diffuse cerebral atrophy with prominent sulci with the coronal view (D) showing greyish pallor of the periventricular white matter consistent with chronic demyelination characteristic of advanced, end-stage MS. Axial views of the postmortem spinal cord demonstrated by T2-weighted MRI obtained *ex situ* (E) shows extensive lesion burden involving both gray and white matter structures, which on histology (F) confirms demyelination (asterix) by immunohistochemistry labeled with the myelin protein, proteo-lipid protein (myelin depicted in brown). The extensive MS lesion burden in both the brain and spinal cord was responsible for the significant, irreversible disability the patient experienced during life.

Suggested Reading

World Health Organization. *World Health Organization Definition of Palliative Care.* www.who.int/cancer/palliative/definition/en/.

Hawley PH. The bow tie model of 21st century palliative care. *J Pain Symptom Manage.* 2014 Jan;**47**(1):e2–5.

Lunde HMB, Assmus J, Myhr KM, Bo L, Grytten N. Survival and cause of death in multiple sclerosis: A 60-year-longitudinal population study. *J Neurol Neurosurg Psychiatry.* 2017 Aug; **88**(8):621–5. Epub 2017 Apr 1.

Strupp J, Romotzky V, Galushko M, Golla H, Voltz R. Palliative care for severely affected patients with multiple sclerosis: When and why? Results of a Delphi survey of health care professionals. *J Palliat Med.* 2014 Oct;**17**(10): 1128–36.

The MS Society: MS and Palliative Care. www.mssociety.org.uk/sites/default/files/Documents/Professionals/MS%20and%20Palliative%20Care%20-%20guide%20for%20professionals.pdf

Veronese S, Gallo G, Valle A, et al. Specialist palliative care improves the quality of life in advanced neurodegenerative disorders: NE-PAL, a pilot randomised controlled study *BMJ Supportive & Palliative Care* Published Online First: July 16, 2015.

Comparing and Contrasting the Approach to Advance Care Planning in Multiple Sclerosis

Aynharan Sinnarajah

Clinical History

A 45-year-old man with a wife and two young children presented to his family physician with a weeks-long history of lower extremity weakness and stiffness. He was eventually diagnosed with primary progressive multiple sclerosis.

His family physician, knowing the incurable nature of this chronic disease, recognized the need to start discussing advance care planning soon, when he still had full cognitive capacity. He gently introduced the topic to the patient and his wife over the course of the next year. They discussed a) what he would wish for, if he were ever unable to speak for himself with poor quality of life, and very little likelihood of recovery (he wanted to shift the focus of his care to comfort only, with no further hospitalizations); b) what he would want, if he were ever unable to eat or drink for himself (he might choose a percutaneous endoscopic gastrostomy tube if his quality of life was still good); and c) where he would want his care when he approached the end of life (he wanted to be at home or in a hospice if his care needs were too high). He documented these wishes in his advance directive and he communicated these wishes to his closest family so that they were aware of them. Even though there were a lot of tears during the discussion, he and his wife were comforted that they could plan for the future on their own terms, rather than in moments of crisis.

Palliative Domain of Care

Structure and Processes of Care – Interdisciplinary team assessment based on patient/family goals of care; prognosis; disposition (level of care – inpatient unit, home); referral to palliative care services to guide decisions about the goals of care
The World Health Organization (WHO) defines palliative care as an approach that improves the quality of life of patients and their families facing the problems associated with life-threatening illness, through the prevention and relief of suffering by means of early identification and impeccable assessment and treatment of pain and other physical, psychosocial, and spiritual problems [1]. It is care that is patient- and family-centered. Multiple sclerosis, being a life-threatening illness, can benefit from a palliative care approach implemented early in the disease course, as outlined in this case. Appropriate attention was paid early to the patient and his family's physical and psychosocial needs, knowing the incurable nature of his disease.

Since palliative care is an approach to care that incorporates attention to quality of life while receiving disease-targeted therapies, it should be offered by any health care professional. *Primary palliative care* is care that can be provided by the family physician (as in this case) and neurology teams. If expert help is needed (e.g., complex symptom management), then specialized palliative care teams can be called in on a consultative basis, to provide *secondary palliative care*. Sometimes, the needs are very complex and the palliative care specialist will need to take over care, with occasional admittance into a hospital palliative care unit to provide *tertiary palliative care*. The neurology and family physicians are still involved to help with the care of the patient.

Ideally, the palliative care approach should start near the beginning of the diagnosis of multiple sclerosis. In the beginning, most of the care will be focused on disease-targeted therapies in the case of active inflammatory disease (as may be seen in relapsing-remitting MS), while palliative care will only be a small part of the overall care. However, as the disease evolves palliative care will become a major part of the care. The bowtie model proposed by Hawley is especially useful to conceptualise this when introducing the topic of palliative care during the early stages of a life-threatening illness (Figures 47.1 and 47.2) [2].

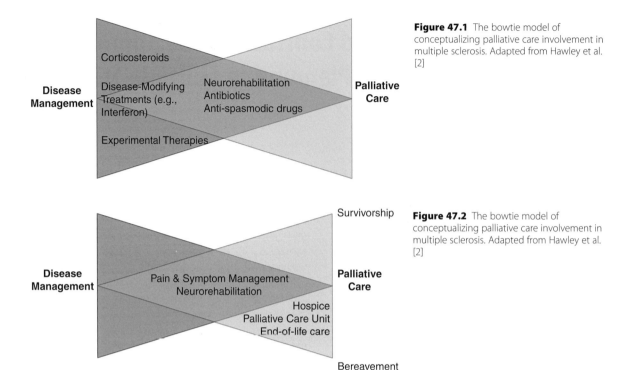

Figure 47.1 The bowtie model of conceptualizing palliative care involvement in multiple sclerosis. Adapted from Hawley et al. [2]

Figure 47.2 The bowtie model of conceptualizing palliative care involvement in multiple sclerosis. Adapted from Hawley et al. [2]

Palliative Care Discussion

Palliative care encompasses end-of-life issues but also includes a patient- and family-centered approach with attention paid to physical, psychosocial, and spiritual dimensions of care at the time of diagnosis of a life-limiting illness. As such, the family physician plays a key role in inquiring about these aspects of care with the patient and family. The neurology team can also play a role by asking about symptoms and referring to appropriate specialists when needed. We also know that patients really value the input of their neurology teams who are the experts in multiple sclerosis, especially around future goal setting and prognosis.

Discussions about coping may elicit feelings of depression and suicidal thoughts associated with MS. If they are recognized early, the patient and family may be able to access needed resources quickly with resulting improvement in their quality of life.

Early advance care planning discussions are valuable to ensure that patients receive goal-concordant care and to reduce the likelihood of major decisions about life-prolonging care needing to be made in crisis situations. This is highlighted by the patient's receipt of care that was consistent with his preferences. Since they had already thought through this, when the end of life approached, there was no crisis and appropriate resources were mobilised to support the patient and family at home.

Clinical Course

After a few years, he started having some pain that impacted his quality of life and function, despite the use of analgesics such as acetaminophen. Small doses of opioids were introduced with careful monitoring. Even though initially he was reluctant to start stronger analgesics, he saw the improvement in his function and quality of life and was glad that he had tried it.

As the years progressed, he continued to decline and his disability was now severe enough to affect his day-to-day care. His pain started increasing as well. He was referred to a palliative care team. A palliative care nurse and physician visited him and his family at home. They reviewed his current symptoms (both physical and psychosocial), functional limitations, and advance care planning documents. His pain medications were adjusted and occupational and physiotherapist referrals were made to assess his home to help with his mobility. They also got access to a 24/7 emergency home care number that he could call anytime for help with symptoms.

The palliative home care team continued to assess him regularly over time. One day, he admitted to suicidal thoughts due to the feelings of being a burden on his family. He was diagnosed with depression, an antidepressant was started, and a home care social worker started seeing him. This was very helpful.

He was now sixty-five and now mostly in bed. His cognition had worsened with increasing periods of somnolence and confusion. The palliative team prepared the family for the approaching end of life. Due to the earlier advance care planning discussions by the patient, the family knew that they were respecting his wishes to keep him at home. Comfort medications through parenteral access route (subcutaneous administration) were made available at home. More nursing support was instituted to support his caregivers as well as for medication administration. His extended family visited him over many days to support his family and be in his presence. He died peacefully with his wife and two children at his bedside.

General Remarks

Multiple sclerosis is a chronic, inflammatory demyelinating disease of the central nervous system with substantial clinical heterogeneity. For some patients, the disease will only manifest as an occasional sensory nuisance over decades while for others it can lead to death within weeks of symptom onset. Given this marked variability in clinical outcome, goals of care need to be highly individualized and frequently revisited.

The greatest determinant of long-term disability in multiple sclerosis is entry into the progressive phase. As the disease can affect any part of the central nervous system, the myriad of symptoms a patient can experience is broad, ranging from weakness, spasticity, ataxia, and sensory alterations (such as numbness, paresthesias, and pain) to sphincteric disturbance (such as urinary and bowel dysfunction), visual troubles (such as poor acuity and diplopia), bulbar symptoms (such as dysphagia and dysarthria), language difficulties, cognitive decline, and fatigue, among others. These symptoms can be debilitating and lead to secondary complications as in the patient discussed in the previous chapter who experienced recurrent infections related to her severe immobility and poor sphincteric function. Cognitive impairment is common, can occur early in the disease, and can have an enormously deleterious impact on quality of life. Despite this, cognitive dysfunction in MS is often under-recognized and under-diagnosed. In a chronic disease with evolving care needs, this is problematic,

especially when discussions about goals of care and end-of-life care are left too late, when the patient can no longer meaningfully contribute. As in this case, it's often better to have these discussions early in the course of the disease. Life expectancy in MS is reduced by almost a decade compared to the general population, making these discussions all the more relevant [3].

The mobilization of palliative care pathways early in the course of the disease can help inform decision-making and patient care goals (thereby avoiding family conflict) but also coordinate symptom management, as exemplified in the case discussed in this chapter. In the case featured in the previous chapter, the patient had a long-standing history of constipation suboptimally managed by several health care providers. She had been constipated for a week prior to the current admission. This is particularly salient in that case as she had a documented history of constipation "splinting" her diaphragm, causing her to develop atelectasis and then pneumonia. Her severe spasticity and poor mobility undoubtedly were contributing factors and yet her spasticity continued to worsen despite baclofen and regular Botox injections, again managed by different health care providers. A several-year history of dysphagia likely contributed to recurrent aspiration and yet a PEG tube was only considered at the very end stage of her disease. In contrast, earlier discussions of PEG options led to a community focused management of end-of-life care in the case covered in this chapter. A coordinated care approach offered by a family physician and a palliative care service improved the management of these complex symptoms while providing regular guidance about decision-making related to goals of care.

General Conclusions

Multiple sclerosis is a chronic disease with striking clinical heterogeneity in clinical outcome. People with MS can have a wide range of evolving symptoms, many disabling, that require ongoing and coordinated input of several health care professionals across a diverse range of specialties and expertise. Goals of care need to be addressed early in the course of the disease, even when the patient demonstrates minimal "overt" disability. Health care providers need to be aware of the prevalence and impact of cognitive dysfunction in MS to ensure that people with MS are meaningfully involved in discussions about these goals of care for symptom management and end-of-life care at an early stage of their disease. As MS typically affects younger people during the productive years of life, the involvement of palliative care early on in the course of the disease is often seen as taboo by both patients and health care providers and therefore, neglected. Increased awareness about the scope of palliative care in this patient group is urgently needed. Focusing on what the patient and family needs are at all stages of their disease can be good way to ensure a palliative approach alongside their disease-targeted therapies. After all, early involvement of palliative care can facilitate appropriate, coordinated symptom management, caregiver support, transitions in care, and advance care planning, which has considerable benefit to patients with MS and their families.

Suggested Reading

1. World Health Organization. *World Health Organization Definition of Palliative Care.* www.who.int/cancer/palliative/definition/en/

2. Hawley PH. The bow tie model of 21st century palliative care. *J Pain Symptom Manage.* 2014 Jan;**47**(1):e2–5.

3. Lunde HMB, Assmus J, Myhr KM, Bo L, Grytten N. Survival and cause of death in multiple sclerosis: A 60-year-longitudinal population study. *J Neurol Neurosurg Psychiatry.* 2017 Aug; **88**(8):621–5. Epub 2017 Apr 1.

4. Strupp J, Romotzky V, Galushko M, Golla H, Voltz R. Palliative care for severely affected patients with multiple sclerosis: When and why? Results of a Delphi survey of health care professionals. *J Palliat Med.* 2014 Oct;**17**(10):1128–36.

5. The MS Society: MS and Palliative Care. www.mssociety.org.uk/sites/default/files/Documents/Professionals/MS%20and%20Palliative%20Care%20-%20guide%20for%20professionals.pdf

6. Veronese S, Gallo G, Valle A, et al. Specialist palliative care improves the quality of life in advanced neurodegenerative disorders: NE-PAL, a pilot randomised controlled study *BMJ Supportive & Palliative Care.* Published Online First: July 16, 2015.

Chapter 48

Neuropsychological Disturbances and Fatigue in Multiple Sclerosis

A. Sebastian Lopez-Chiriboga

Clinical History

A 22-year-old right-handed Caucasian woman was admitted to the neurology service for evaluation of new onset diplopia and right-sided hemiparesis. These new symptoms were preceded by an episode of bilateral lower extremity sensory loss and gait imbalance, leading to frequent falls that improved spontaneously two months prior to her admission.

Before her hospitalization, she was seen locally by an ophthalmologist who recommended MRI imaging of the brain for further evaluation. This study showed evidence of multifocal brain enhancing and non-enhancing lesions, and a local neurologist recommended high doses of oral prednisone for five days. She presented to our emergency department after there was no significant improvement with oral steroids.

Examination

Vital Signs: Blood Pressure 110/70 mmHg afebrile, Heart Rate: 80 beats per minute, Respiratory Rate: 18

The neurological examination was pertinent for decreased attention but otherwise she had a normal mental status exam. Her cranial nerve examination revealed normal gaze in primary position, left impaired adduction with nystagmus in the right eye on right gaze and normal left abduction on left gaze. No afferent pupillary defect was found, and the remainder of the cranial nerve exam was normal. The motor examination was consistent with an upper motor neuron pattern of weakness affecting the right upper and lower extremities 4/5.

She had hyperreflexia with an extensor plantar response on the right.

Sensory loss was noted in the lower extremities to pinprick and she had a sensory level at T7.

She had right upper extremity ataxia and an ataxic gait with a positive Romberg sign.

Inpatient Evaluation

During her hospitalization, an MRI brain with and without gadolinium and an MRI of the thoracic cord (Figure 48.1) revealed multiple foci of abnormal signal consistent with prior and new areas of demyelination in multiple regions.

An extensive laboratory evaluation for rheumatologic, lymphoproliferative and infectious disorders was negative. A cerebrospinal fluid analysis showed: red blood cells < 3,000; white blood cells 11; Neutrophils 25 percent; glucose 85; protein 18, RPR, Viral PCRs (Negative), Aquaporin 4 (AQP4) IgG Serum/CSF: Negative, MOG IgG: Negative, Oligoclonal bands: 10. IgG Index: Elevated 0.91, JC Virus Ab: Negative.

The classic imaging findings and clinical features were consistent with relapsing remitting multiple sclerosis (MS); the diagnosis was discussed with her and she experienced significant anxiety due to the chronic and possibly severely disabling and relapsing nature of her condition.

She was treated with IV methylprednisolone 1 gram daily for five days and her neurologic deficits started to improve. She was subsequently transferred to an inpatient rehabilitation facility.

Palliative Domains of Care

Physical Aspects of Care – Acute decline in performance status, fatigue

Psychological and Social Aspects of Care – Coping with chronic illness

She was an otherwise very healthy young woman who was recently engaged. She was in the process of planning her wedding and finishing a degree in advertising. Her neurologic deficits prevented her from performing her usual activities of daily living and they necessitated temporary withdrawal from college, causing a significant amount of stress and uncertainty. Although her family and her fiancé were very

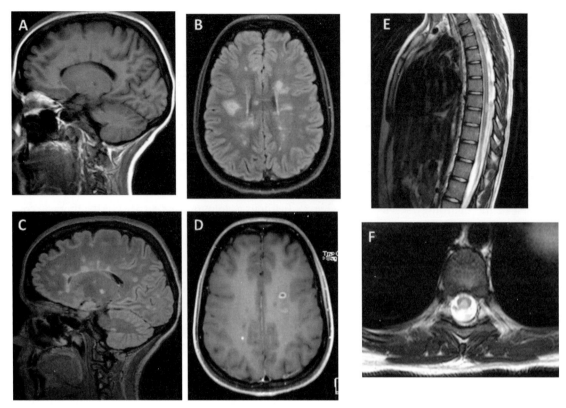

Figure 48.1 Multiple foci of abnormal signal intensity within the cerebral white matter bilaterally, including the periventricular, juxtacortical and deep cerebral white matter bilaterally; the corpus callosum; the posterior limb of the left internal capsule the right pontomedullary junction; and the left middle cerebellar peduncle (B–C). Many of the foci demonstrated decreased T1 signal intensity (A) some demonstrate abnormal ring like enhancement (D). MRI of the thoracic spine showed two unenhancing oval-shaped T2 hyperintense plaque-like lesions within the thoracic cord, extending from the mid-T8 vertebral body to the top of T9 vertebral body (E–F).

supportive, she worried about being a burden to her future husband and to her family. Coping with a diagnosis of multiple sclerosis was very difficult for her and her family due to the rapidly progressive deficits affecting her neurologic system and the potential consequences of the disease on her future career and family. When contemplating a pregnancy, the choice of a disease-modifying drug is important. In this case, due to the significant clinical and radiographic disease activity, natalizumab was recommended, delaying her plans of starting a family.

Palliative Care Discussion

After reviewing the MRI findings [1] and clinical history, she received a diagnosis of relapsing remitting multiple sclerosis [2]. Discussing the diagnosis of a chronic illness such as multiple sclerosis can be difficult for physicians and receiving the diagnosis of a chronic and potentially severely debilitating

neurologic disorder can cause a tremendous amount of distress in patients [3].

Helping patients cope with their disease is crucial at this stage. A detailed explanation of the pathophysiology of the condition and the current therapeutic strategies is helpful to decrease anxiety and to provide hope for the patient with a new diagnosis of multiple sclerosis. A palliative approach to care that focuses on the whole person and not just on the disease itself is appropriate for all patients with multiple sclerosis, which is a chronic and progressive disease. Addressing the physical, psychological, social, and spiritual aspects of care is necessary to ensure that the needs of patients are being met.

Clinical Course

Four weeks after her hospital discharge, she returned for her follow-up visit. After the administration of IV steroids and intensive rehabilitation, her symptoms improved significantly. She had residual minor diplopia on left gaze and she was able to walk without assistive devices.

She developed significant fatigue, affecting her ability to continue with college, that failed to respond to methylphenidate and amantadine.

Due to the significant amount of disease activity, the radiographic findings, and considering her JC virus antibody negative status, initiation of highly effective therapy with natalizumab was recommended. She was considering having children shortly after her wedding. However, due to the recent diagnosis of multiple sclerosis and the disease-modifying agent, she was counseled that she would not be able to achieve that goal within the expected time frame.

General Remarks

Living with multiple sclerosis can be challenging and introducing palliative care early in the disease process can be very beneficial. Palliative care can assist with the evaluation and management of certain symptoms such as complex and chronic pain, coping with the disease, and mood disorders [4, 5]. Family and caregiver burden can also be addressed.

The management of fatigue in MS patients is challenging, as the pathophysiology is complex and usually multifactorial [6]. Amantadine, modafinil, and armodafinil are commonly prescribed medications for fatigue but they are rarely associated with a complete response. The management of fatigue in MS is multidisciplinary and it includes energy conservation strategies, cooling devices, cognitive behavioral therapy in combination with medications, and

appropriate management of comorbid disorders that can also contribute to fatigue.

The decline in her performance status and the disruption in her exciting life plans (marriage, graduation, possible pregnancy) caused a significant amount of distress, anxiety, and frustration. Neuropsychiatric symptoms are frequent in the MS population [7] and they should be recognized early and treated with non-pharmacologic and pharmacologic strategies as deemed necessary.

Suggested Reading

1. Filippi, M, et al., MRI criteria for the diagnosis of multiple sclerosis: MAGNIMS consensus guidelines. *Lancet Neurol.* 2016;**15**(3):292–303.

2. Polman, CH, et al., Diagnostic criteria for multiple sclerosis: 2010 revisions to the McDonald criteria. *Ann Neurol.* 2011;**69**(2):292–302.

3. Golla, H., et al., Multiple sclerosis and palliative care – perceptions of severely affected multiple sclerosis patients and their health professionals: A qualitative study. *BMC Palliat Care.* 2014;**13**(1):11.

4. Strupp J, Voltz R, Golla H. Opening locked doors: Integrating a palliative care approach into the management of patients with severe multiple sclerosis. *Mult Scler.* 2016 Jan;**22**(1):13–18. Epub 2015 Oct 7.

5. Vanopdenbosch LJ, Oliver DJ, Kass JS. Palliative care in multiple sclerosis. *Continuum.* 2016 Aug;**22**(3):943–6.

6. Braley, TJ, Chervin, RD. Fatigue in multiple sclerosis: Mechanisms, evaluation, and treatment. *Sleep.* 2010; **33**(8):1061–7.

7. Figved, N., et al., Neuropsychiatric symptoms in patients with multiple sclerosis. *Acta Psychiatr Scand.* 2005;**112**(6):463–8.

Pain and Psychosocial Symptoms in Newly Diagnosed Neuromyelitis Optica Spectrum Disorder (NMOSD)

A. Sebastian Lopez-Chiriboga

Clinical History

A 46-year-old right-handed African-American woman with a history of systemic lupus erythematosus (SLE) suffered an episode of right retroorbital pain and vision loss; she was diagnosed with right-sided optic neuritis after an MR brain revealed T2 hyperintensities and gadolinium enhancement in the right optic nerve (Figure 49.1). She received intravenous methylprednisolone with subsequent improvement of her symptoms. Approximately three weeks later, she developed intractable nausea, vomiting, and hiccups followed by bilateral upper and lower extremity weakness that rapidly progressed to paraplegia. She also experienced urinary retention, requiring the placement of an indwelling urinary catheter, and prominent thoracic back pain.

An MRI of the spine with and without gadolinium demonstrated a longitudinally extensive lesion starting at C-5 extending to the inferior aspect of T10 with patchy enhancement (Figure 49.2).

A lumbar puncture was performed and cerebrospinal fluid analysis revealed evidence of a lymphocytic pleocytosis: Total nucleated cells (TNC) 40, 70 percent lymphocytes, protein 85 mg/dL (normal less than 45 mg/dL), normal glucose; viral polymerase chain reactions, gram stain, and bacterial cultures were negative. Aquaporin 4 (QP4) Ig-G was positive in the serum. She was diagnosed with Neuromyelitis Optica Spectrum Disorder (NMOSD) – AQP4 positive according to the 2015 criteria [1].

She was treated with IV methylprednisolone 1,000 mg daily for five days and mild improvement of the upper extremity weakness was noted. However, she remained paraplegic. Plasmapheresis was initiated with minimal improvement in her lower extremity strength and rituximab was administered prior to her discharge to rehabilitation. During her hospitalization, her

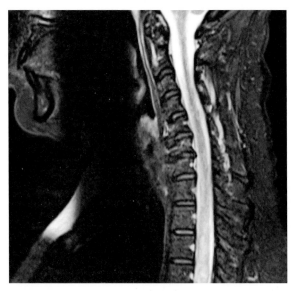

Figure 49.2 A) MRI cervical spine shows a longitudinally extensive T2 hyperintense lesion affecting several levels starting at C5 extending to T10.
B) MR Thoracic spine axial view reveals a T2 hyperintense centrally located expansile lesion.

Figure 49.1 MR brain with and without gadolinium. T2 hyperintensities and optic nerve edema and gadolinium enhancement.

nausea and vomiting were very difficult to control, requiring multiple doses of antiemetic drugs with moderate response. She was subsequently very frustrated, anxious, and tearful due to the acute neurologic decline.

Examination

Vital Signs: Blood pressure 120/75 mmHg afebrile, Heart rate: 98 beats per minute, Respiratory rate: 18

She had a right afferent pupillary defect, vision was 20/60 on the right 20/20 on the left, and the remainder of the cranial nerve examination was normal.

There was decreased arm abduction right greater than left and no effort against gravity in the lower extremities. She had decreased reflexes in the upper extremities and absent patellar reflexes. A sensory level was approximately at T9. Vibration and proprioception were absent in the lower extremities and decreased in the upper extremities.

Palliative Domains of Care

Physical Aspects of Care – Significant acute decline in performance status

She had a major decline in her performance status. She was previously healthy, and within four weeks she became dependent in most of her activities of daily living, including basic mobility and transfer. She also lost urinary control and required an indwelling catheter placement.

Psychological Aspects of Care – Anxiety, depression

Due to the acute decline in her ability to function, she began experiencing multiple psychiatric symptoms, including reactional anxiety, frustration, and fear, due to the uncertainty of her prognosis and future functional status.

Palliative Care Discussion

This patient had no prior history of psychiatric disorders and she enjoyed her quality of life prior to this hospitalization. After receiving a diagnosis of NMOSD with AQP4-IgG, she demonstrated difficulty coping with her functional limitations. She developed severe paraparesis and urinary retention, reducing her mobility. She also experienced intractable nausea and vomiting related to her diagnosis, which can be a challenging symptom to treat [2]. Her physical symptoms impaired her ability to perform her activities of daily living, causing her to be more reliant on

others, and the loss of independence was difficult to accept. The life that she knew was no longer her reality and the realization of her new condition led to emotional and psychological distress. The frustration and uncertainty regarding the degree of residual disability caused anxiety and a low mood.

Clinical Course

One week after her hospital discharge she began recovering motor function in the lower extremities. Despite some noticeable improvement in her neurologic status, her progress plateaued as she developed painful spasms affecting the upper extremities bilaterally that occurred multiple times a day and that affected her ability to participate in physical therapy. Diazepam and cyclobenzaprine were initiated without significant benefit and opiates led to cognitive side effects without symptomatic improvement. Four weeks after discharge she was able to ambulate with the assistance of a walker and her bladder dysfunction was managed through intermittent catheterization. Although she was more accepting of her diagnosis, she continued to wonder if she would improve enough function to regain her independence.

General Remarks

She experienced significant morbidity in the setting of a diagnosis of NMOSD. Along with the disabling symptoms, she also developed pain [3] secondary to the inflammatory myelopathy. Her pain was subsequently complicated by paroxysmal tonic spasms. Severe pain is common in patients with transverse myelitis due to NMOSD, which can contribute to the underlying depression and negatively affect their quality of life. Recent studies show that pain in this group of patients is not particularly well managed [4].

The marked decline from her baseline functional status affected her tremendously, causing situational anxiety and likely an adjustment disorder. Approximately 30 percent of patients with NMOSD develop depression and this prevalence is higher than what has been described in the general population [5]. Although it is well described, it is also undertreated [5]. Counseling patients and offering support is crucial when they face a major acute decline in their performance status. Psychiatric and psychological evaluations may also be beneficial. Standardized questionnaires at follow-up visits could be useful to identify potential unmet therapeutic needs in this patient population.

Suggested Reading

1. Wingerchuk DM, Banwell B, Bennett JL, Cabre P, Carroll W, Chitnis T, de Seze J, Fujihara K, Greenberg B, Jacob A, Jarius S, Lana-Peixoto M, Levy M, Simon JH, Tenembaum S, Traboulsee AL, Waters P, Wellik KE, Weinshenker BG. International panel for NMO for neuromyelitis optica diagnosis. International consensus diagnostic criteria for neuromyelitis optica spectrum disorders. *Neurology*. 2015 Jul 14;**85**(2):177–89.

2. Iorio R, Lucchinetti CF, Lennon VA, Farrugia G, Pasricha PJ, Weinshenker BG, Pittock SJ. Intractable nausea and vomiting from autoantibodies against a brain water channel. *Clin Gastroenterol Hepatol*. 2013 Mar;**11**(3):240–5.

3. Kanamori Y, Nakashima I, Takai Y, Nishiyama S, Kuroda H, Takahashi T, Kanaoka-Suzuki C, Misu T, Fujihara K, Itoyama Y. Pain in neuromyelitis optica and its effect on quality of life: A cross-sectional study. *Neurology*. 2011 Aug 16;**77**(7):652–8.

4. Kong Y, Okoruwa H, Revis J, Tackley G, Leite MI, Lee M, Tracey I, Palace J. Pain in patients with transverse myelitis and its relationship to aquaporin 4 antibody status. *J Neurol Sci*. 2016 Sep 15;**368**:84–8.

5. Chavarro VS, Mealy MA, Simpson A, Lacheta A, Pache F, Ruprecht K, Gold SM, Paul F, Brandt AU, Levy M. Insufficient treatment of severe depression in neuromyelitis optica spectrum disorder. *Neurol Neuroimmunol Neuroinflamm*. 2016 Oct 24;**3**(6):e286.

Index